Fringe Electronic

"Medical" Devices

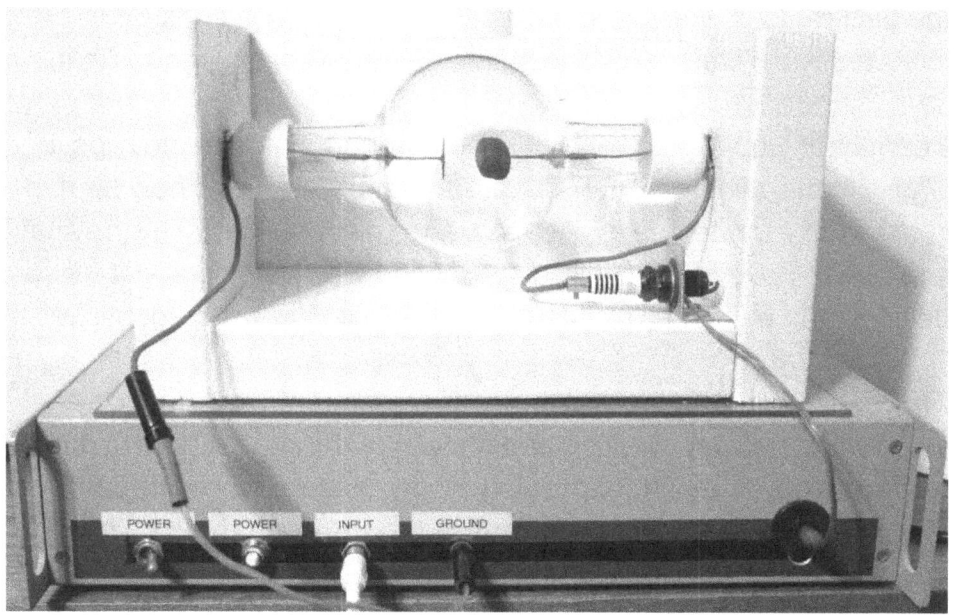

By Robert J Davis II

Fringe Electronic "Medical" Devices (and some not so medical)
By Robert J Davis II, Copyright 2012, 2014, 2021

Introduction

This is an expanded version that now includes some devices that are not necessarily "medical" in nature. My experimenting with these devices grew out of my research into the "medical" devices.

Fringe medical electronics has been around for a long time. They have developed a reputation for being total quackery. The first such device that I heard of was when someone asked me for a picture of my sick daughter. He wanted to put the picture into his machine, to see what treatments she needed. I knew that any analysis of a picture would only come up with the chemicals that the picture itself was made out of. That would be like taking a picture of your car to your mechanic, to see what is wrong with it.

Years later when I was reintroduced to fringe "medical" devices it was with a brochure about "Royal Raymond Rife", and how he had successfully treated several cases of terminal cancer. This device seemed to have a basis in reality. Soon I was reading about these devices and building all kinds of these devices to experiment with.

This book is an attempt at documenting some of these fringe electronic "medical" devices and show you the reader how to build them and how they might possibly work. **None of the devices in this book are in anyway guaranteed to cure anything!** This book is just for someone who wants to experiment or to see what has been tried over the years.

Disclaimer: None of these devices are approved for the treatment of any medical condition. Most of these devices can be very unsafe to build, use or to operate. Anyone with any internal wiring such as a pacemaker must not go anywhere near these devices as serious injury or death may result! The reader or builder takes any and all responsibility for safely building and or operating these devices.

Chapters:

"Medical" devices

Not so "Medical" devices

Chapter 1

How I got Involved

in Building These Devices.

One day while I was walking between some buildings at work I was in so much pain that I just had to sit down. My legs hurt so much that I could not take another step. A friend who was walking with me told me that I might have something like Lime disease. I told him that if that was the case then I would be in a wheel chair. However soon after that I looked at a lime disease brochure and discovered that not everyone who has lime disease is crippled in a wheelchair.

Then I remembered that back in 1978 I had traveled with some friends from Virginia to another friends wedding in Massachusetts. While we were on the way back home, their car broke down just after we had entered the state of Connecticut. When I remembered that trip I quickly checked the map and discovered that we were most likely in Lime Connecticut! While the guys tried to fix their car I wandered off and picked some raspberries. In the process of picking raspberries I slightly scratched my left wrist.

Back at work someone told me that a doctor should look at the scratch on my wrist. So I went to the doctor and he used some tweezers to remove part of the scab. After close examining he said that it was a tick because it had tiny legs and then he tried to show me the legs. It was so tiny that it was impossible for me to see any legs.

About two or three weeks later I was back at the same doctor's office once again because there was a ring of rash forming on my left wrist. The rash was diagnosed by the doctor as ringworm, and he gave me some topical cream to treat it. A few weeks later I was almost kicked out of the Navy. At my yearly physical there was a one foot round ring shaped rash visible on my back. They used a mirror to show it to me. Soon after that, I was also diagnosed with "poly-arthralgia" that is "multiple pains" and is likely an older term for what is called fibromyalgia today.

My health had slowly deteriorated over about 15 years, and most likely it was from the tick bite that had occurred years ago. I tried everything that I could think of to treat it, and the doctors tried several antibiotics.

Then a friend dropped off a few papers on some electronic medical devices that someone had given them. Since I had built many electronics devices over the years, I started building the devices and testing them out on myself. Eventually I did get better, thanks to using these devices and to taking antibiotics.

Recently I thought that I would put together this book to cover these electronic devices, and show pictures and schematics of them so others can build them as well.

What worked best for me? Well the "Super Thumper" is my number one favorite device. Next up is the "Doug coil", it has a similar effect but it covers a much larger area for faster treatment. Also the "Kirlian plate zapper" is great for giving a boost to your immune system.

I also recommend that you take some sort of natural antibiotics to prevent infections, if you are prone to them. There are over the counter antibiotics out there like tonic water (some claim that quinine is even anti-viral), garlic (eat a clove or take the pills) and vitamin C. I prefer Vitamin C with rose hips, its natural vitamin C.

Chapter 2

How these devices might work.

There is some "science" behind how some of these devices might work. According to some researchers, everything that exists has a "frequency". For instance, a 24 KC signal of sufficient amplitude applied to multiple ultrasonic transducers can cause water to break down into hydrogen and oxygen and then ignite. That process produces a light in the middle of a glass of water! That process is called "sono-luminescence" by scientists and has been reproduced in many science labs. Articles about sono-luminescence can also be found in many science books.

Taking that thought a step further, some say that there are frequencies that can also destroy things like bacteria, viruses and perhaps the right frequency can even destroy cancer. The effective frequency might have something to do with the length of their DNA. That is because DNA is essentially a "coil" and all coils will have a resonant frequency. So by hitting that resonant frequency with enough power you could then, in theory, destroy their DNA.

Cancer might also be targeted in another way. Cancer absorbs more iron that normal healthy tissue does. As we know, iron is highly sensitive to a magnetic field. It might be possible that someone with cancer could take lots of vitamin pills that are high in iron. Then you could treat the iron rich cancer cells with powerful magnetic fields. Hence it is theoretically possible to also target cancer using any type of magnetic field in general, as well as using specific frequencies to target the cancer DNA.

Malaria also has a high sensitivity to magnetic fields in general. As the malaria eats the red blood cells in the blood, it has no method to process the iron that is in those red blood cells. As a result, the iron builds up in large "clumps" inside of the adult malaria cells. This leaves them subject to magnetic fields that can then cause the iron to vibrate, rotate, as well as to heat up. These reactions to magnetic fields may well eventually destroy the malaria.

This information was documented by Washington State University years ago. However as far as I know, no clinical trials have ever been done to determine how effective this treatment would be in the field. At one point I tried to send some magnetic mattress pads to Africa to see if patients got better faster when they used the magnetic mattress pads. I do not know if they even made it there or if they helped at all.

Chapter 3

Hulda Clark

Handheld Devices.

In her book "The Cure for all Diseases" Hulda Clark introduced her electronic treatment device. It is basically a 555 timer IC producing a 32KC square wave output. The output then goes to two copper rods that you hold in your hands. It is thought that the small electric current might produce an effect that is called Electrophoresis. That process opens up the "pores" in cells to be able to more easily receive chemicals, as well as to get rid of unwanted chemicals.

My improved version of her device uses a 4060 crystal controlled oscillator instead. It starts with 32KC and then it divides that frequency all the way down to a frequency of two cycles per second. A 12 position rotary switch allows you to select the frequency that you want to use.

My improved zapper also has the ability to select either 9 or 18 volts from two batteries to power it. An optional LED that is placed in series with a 1 K resistor on the 2 Hz output will tell you if it is working properly. The outputs go to two five inch pieces of 1/2 inch diameter copper pipe that you can hold in your hands. The copper pipes are connected to the zapper via some short jumper wires with alligator clips on their ends.

Here is a parts list to make the zapper.
1 - 4060 IC and socket

2 - 12pf ceramic capacitors
1 – 470K ¼ watt resistor
1 – 1 Meg ¼ watt resistor
1 – 10K variable resistor
2 – 9 volt batteries and battery clips
1 – 3 position power switch
1 – 12 position rotary switch
2 – 5 inch long ½ inch diameter copper pipes
2 – Jumper wires with alligator clips

Below is the schematic diagram of my improved zapper. There are two tiny 12 pf capacitors located one on each side of the 32.768 KC crystal. Also, the 4060 IC does not have a "16" Hertz output, so I do not know why I labeled that switch position.

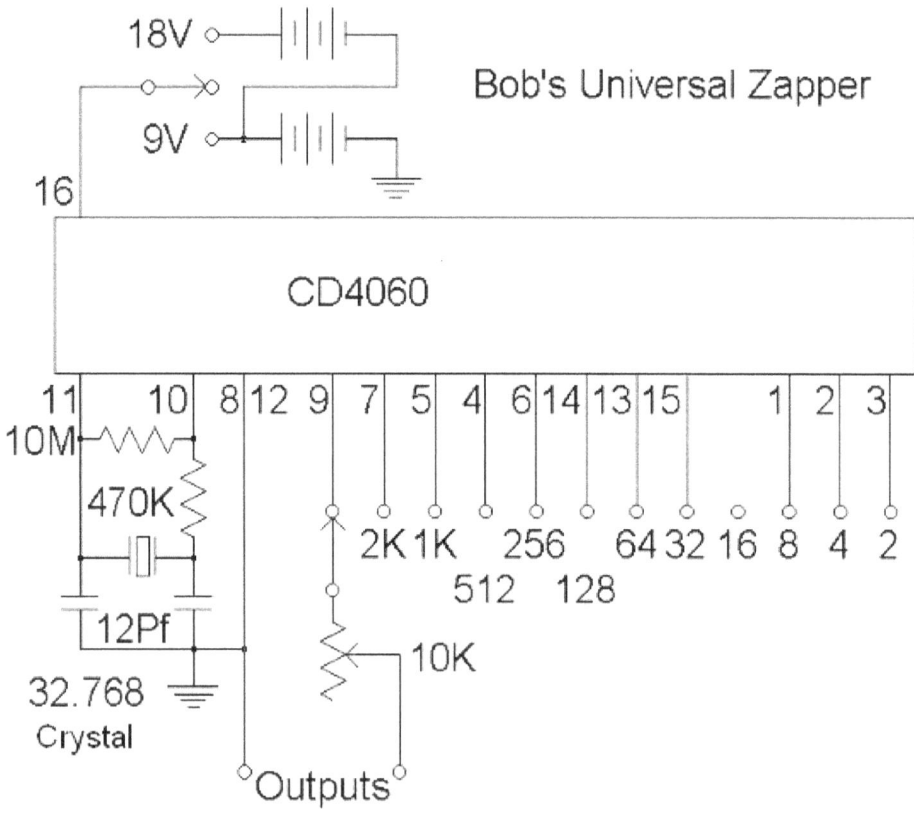

The next picture is what the assembled prototype of my zapping device looks like. I squeezed it all into a small used plastic box. Above the green 12 position switch is a LED that blinks at 2 cycles to let you know the zapper is on and working. That LED was left out of the schematic diagram. The LED needs a 2K to 5K resistor in series with it and connects to the "2" output. You can also see the two nine volt batteries and the yellow power switch that selects between 9V, off, and 18V operation.

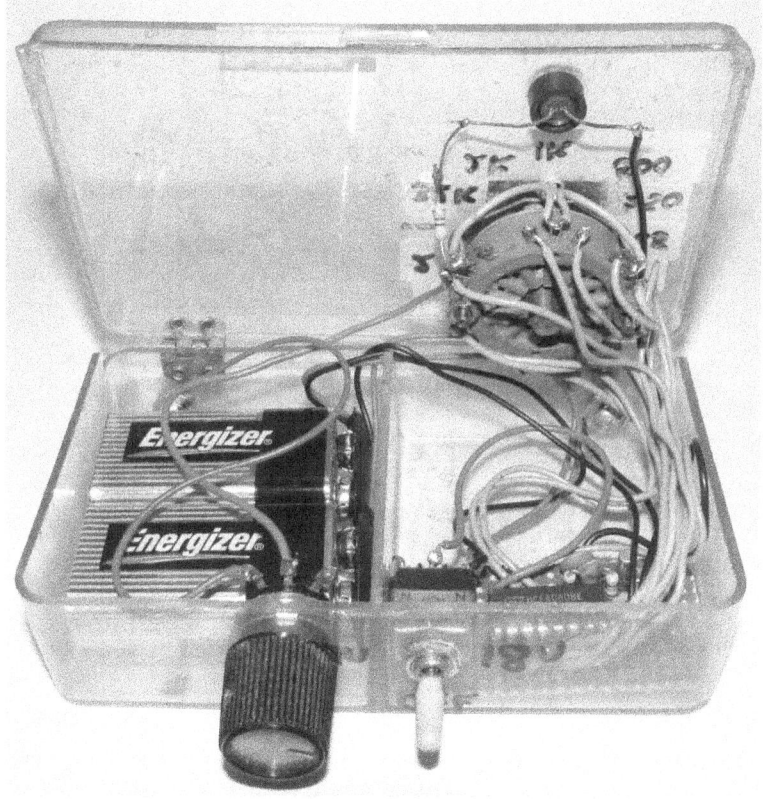

This next picture is a close up of the circuit board showing the 4060 IC chip.

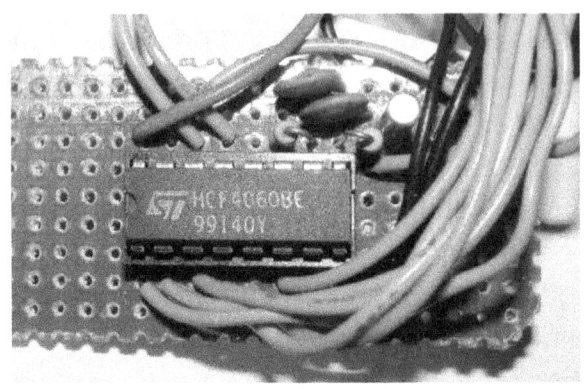

On the next page there is a picture showing the outside view of the Clark like zapper.

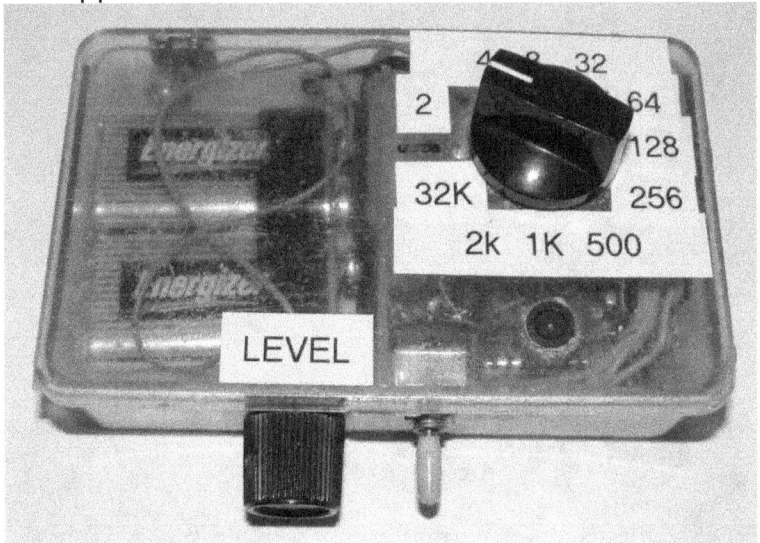

To use this device you will need two jumpers with alligator clips on their ends and two pieces of copper pipe about six inches long. The jumper wires are used to connect the outputs to the copper pipe pieces. You hole one copper pipe piece in each hand and adjust the current to where you can just so feel the pulses.

Chapter 4

Bob Beck,

Pulsed Magnetic Field Device

Bob Beck is know to have developed two devices; one was a hand held electrophoresis device using a relay. It was very similar in operation to the Hulda Clark device, except that it operated at 4 cycles instead of at 32 KC. My device that was shown in the last chapter can produce the 4 Hz output as well. So it can be used as a Hulda Clark device or as a Bob Beck device.

The second Beck device is a pulsed electromagnetic device based on a camera strobe. Basically a coil is placed in series with the strobe's xenon flash tube. You can get a good strobe to use in your experiments from an old fire alarm system or from an old camera.

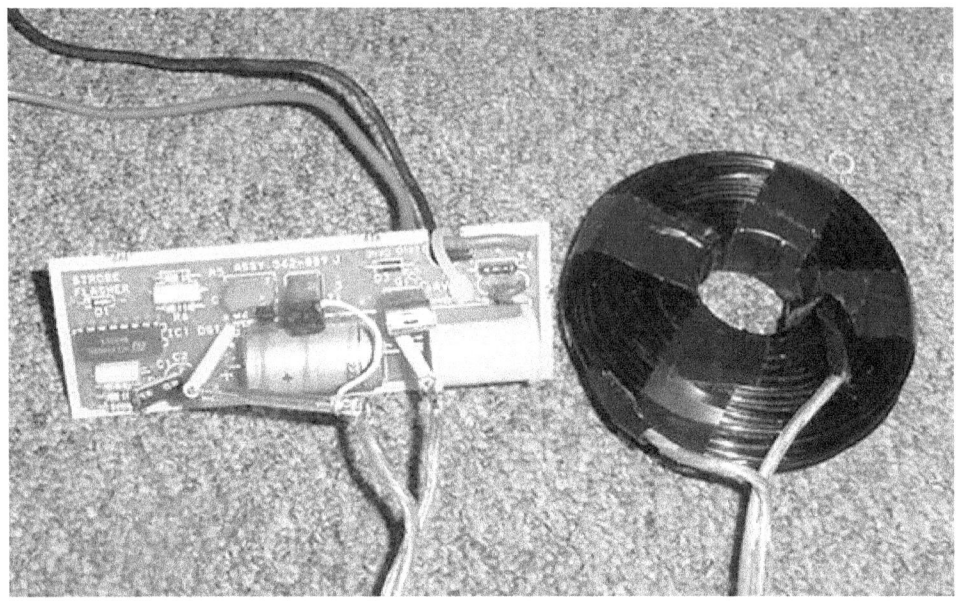

The thumper's electromagnetic coil is made from about 50 feet of 14 gauge enameled wire wound on a reel removed from an old VHS video tape. The reel has to be reinforced or it will bust apart when trying to wind the coil on it. Since the flash runs from an AC adapter, or from batteries, a lot of insulation is not necessary. I have long since upgraded my coil winding form one made with two four to five inch square pieces of plywood. There is about three quarters of an inch length of a one inch in diameter dowel in the middle.

The camera strobe can be replaced with a big SCR to make a much more powerful device. In the picture below the SCR is the device in the upper left hand corner. This big SCR has to handle about 100 amps at 350 volts. I call my device a "Super Thumper". The super thumper uses several 220 to 470 uF at 400 volt capacitors in parallel for about 3200 uF of total capacitance. When this thumper fires it releases about 120 joules of energy into the coil. This can launch a three inch aluminum washer (a hard drive platter works fine) about three to four feet vertically.

The power supply, that is used, consists of a voltage multiplier consisting of 220 uF at 100 volt DC capacitors and 400 volt six amp bridge rectifiers. The SCR is a 1538A73H05 or equivalent. I have no idea what its exact specifications are. However, if the connections to the SCR accidentally come loose, it will throw lots of sparks that fly for a few feet!!

Here is a picture of what it all looks like when it is stuffed into a box that is about 10 inches by eight inches in size. The one meg ohm resistor was replaced with three 330K resistors in series in the picture.

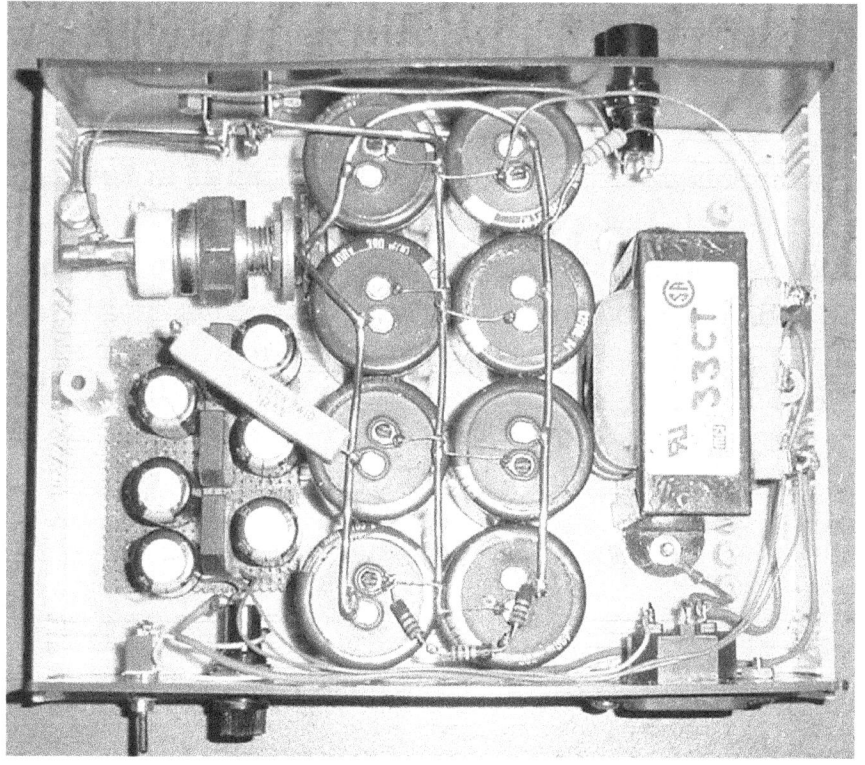

Below is a picture of a completed "Super Thumper" like the many that I have sold on eBay.

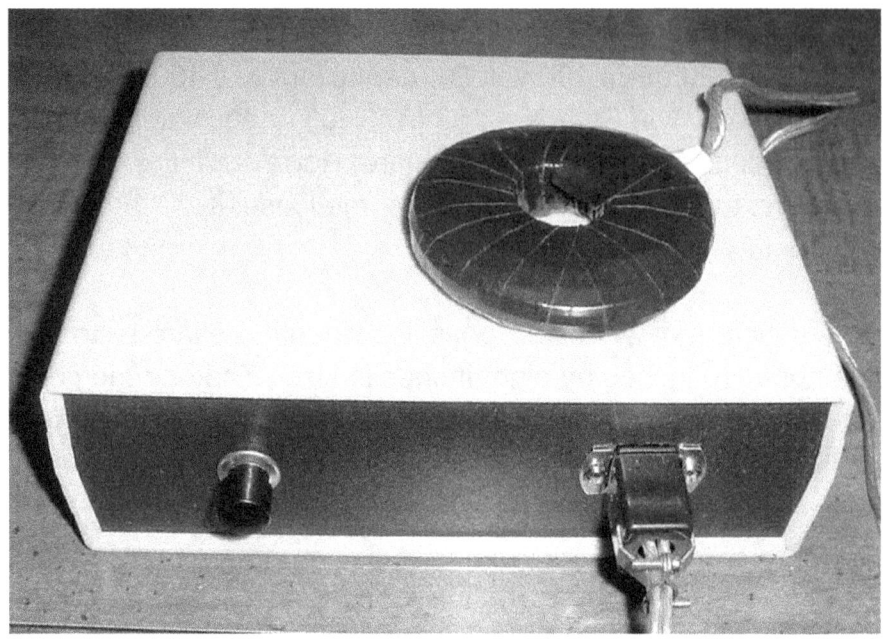

Here is the schematic of the super thumper configured for a transformer that delivers 33-36 volts AC input. For a 25 VAC transformer, use an 8x voltage multiplier. The 10 ohm resistor protects the power supply from being shorted out and must be able to handle about 10 watts. Do not forget to have a 2 amp fuse on the input.

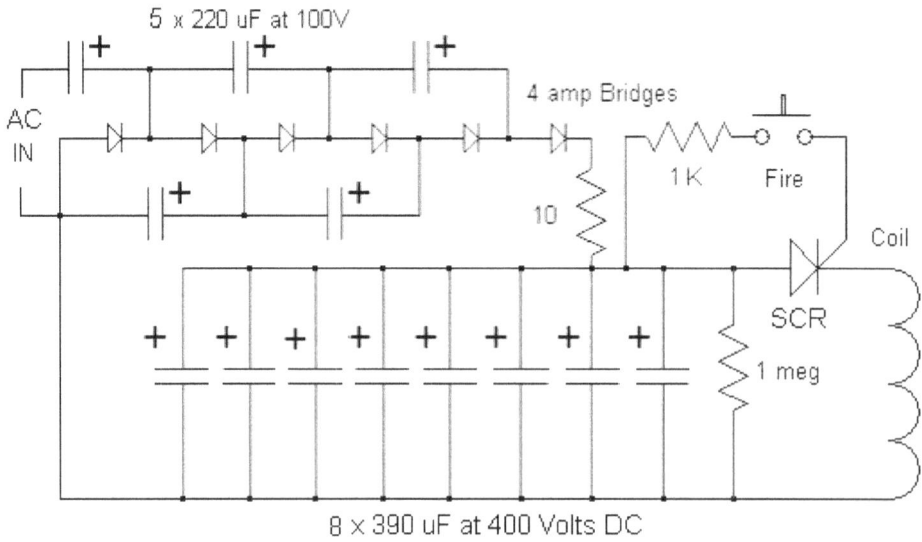

Here is a parts list to build a super thumper.

1 – 35 Volt at 2 amp power transformer
3 – 400 volt at 4 amp bridge rectifiers
1 – 2 Amp fuse and fuse holder
1 – 10 ohm 10 watt resistor
1 – 1 K ohm ½ watt resistor
1 – 1 meg ohm ½ watt resistor
1 – Really big SCR
1 – Momentary contact push button switch
5 – 220 uF at 100 volt capacitors
8 – 390 uF at 400 volt capacitors
1 – Coil of 50 feet of 14 gauge enameled wire.

This type of device is actually somewhat recognized as effective by the medical establishment. They call their somewhat similar device "RTMS" or "TMS" and that stands for "Rapid Trans-cranial Magnetic Stimulation". It is used to treat depression and migraines. However, in my opinion, it can treat many other types of inflammation. They just have not discovered the many things that it can treat yet.

The RTMS device was developed after several severely depressed people had an MRI to see what might be different about their brains. As a result of having the MRI over half of them either improved dramatically or they were cured. Some of the formerly depressed patients left the MRI laughing and joking! This led to making a device that could simulate the powerful magnetic filed of the MRI, but in a smaller device.

Chapter 5

Doug Coil,

Fixed Frequency Magnetic Device

Someone who calls himself "Doug" used a 1000 watt QSC amplifier driving a huge electromagnetic coil device to treat lime disease. A capacitor switch box is connected in series with the coil. Adding the capacitors results in about three times as much voltage. The increased voltage results in over four times as much power going through the coil, compared to using an amplifier to directly drive the coil. That is because power is voltage times current. But if you double the voltage you also double the current because current is equal to voltage divided by resistance. By combining those two formulas we discover that Power is voltage squared over resistance.

At first Doug experimented under a microscope, with a much smaller coil, to see what frequencies were most effective. Then he started making these much bigger coils to actually treat diseases.

The "Doug coil" is usually made out of about 500 feet of insulated 12 gauge wire wound around about a one foot diameter form. The Doug coil is the one that is made with the green wire in the picture below. The coil wrapped in black electrical tape is a smaller coil made from 14 gauge enameled wire that I built for comparison purposes.

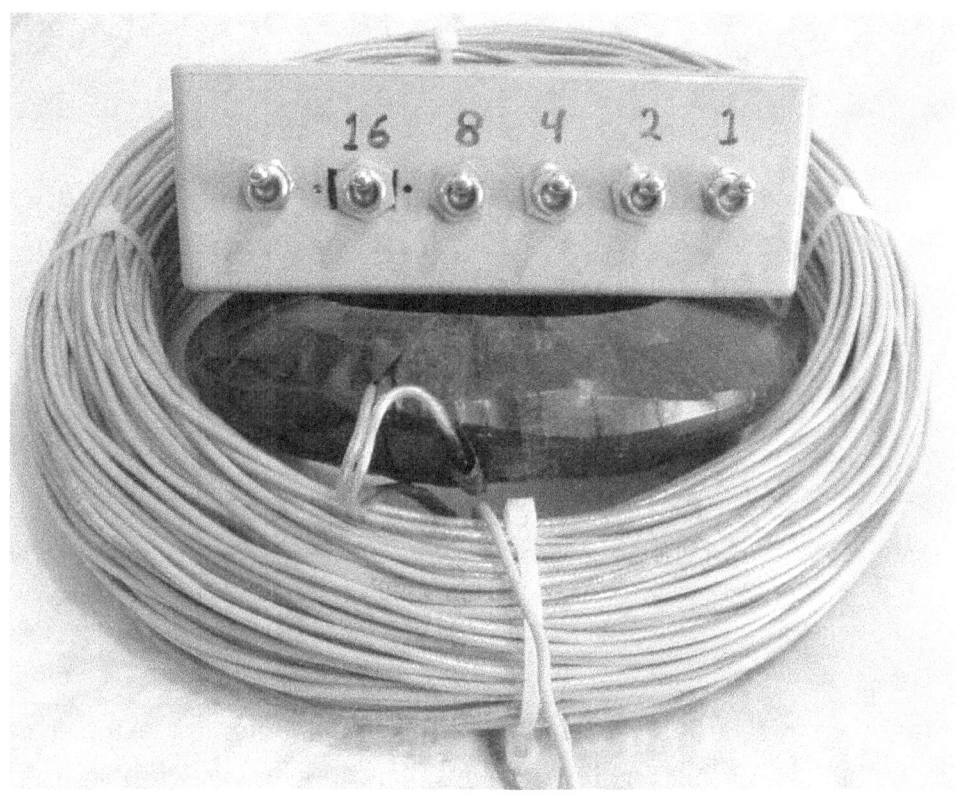

The ultimate test of the power of a Doug coil or any other electromagnet is to make a five inch hard drive platter stand on end. I have tried using 500 feet of 14 gauge enameled wire and it works just as well as the insulated wire does. The insulation creates more space between the wires and that space can actually reduce the strength of the magnetic field that is produced by the coil.

Here is a picture of the 14 gauge enameled wire coil with a five inch aluminum hard drive platter, standing up on one end, from the force of the magnetic field.

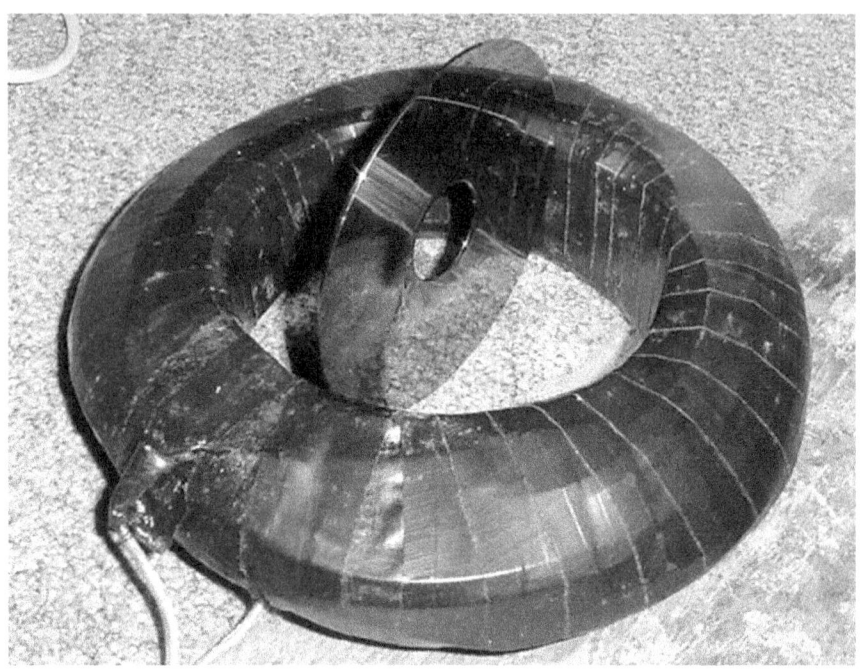

Here is a simplified "schematic" diagram of the Doug coil setup. Everything is "off the shelf" except for the capacitor switch box. This schematic left out the .5uF capacitor and switch. Some switch boxes also have a "bypass" switch.

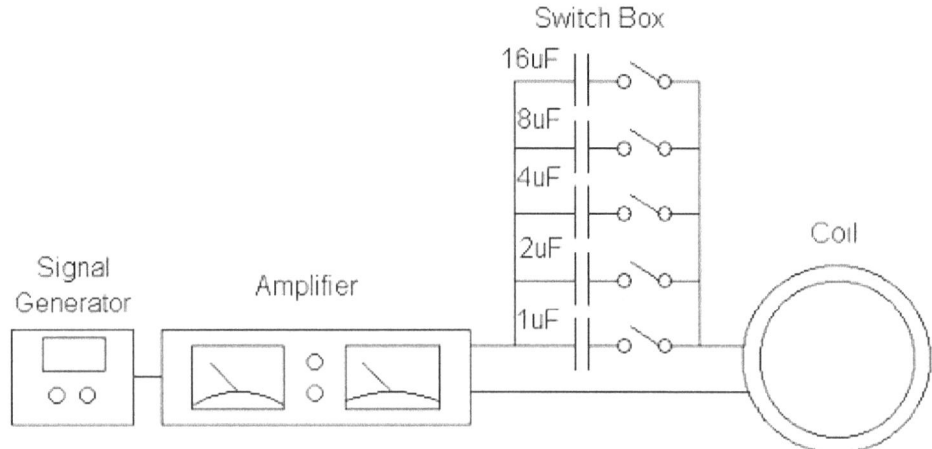

Note that the capacitors in the switch box need to be rated for at least 400 volts AC. Normal 250 volt capacitors will short out and likely fry the amplifier. I am speaking from experience here.

Here is what it looks like inside of a typical capacitor switch box. The many red capacitors on the right are two uF at 400 volts. Two of them are used in series give one uF and in two of them are used in parallel give four uF.

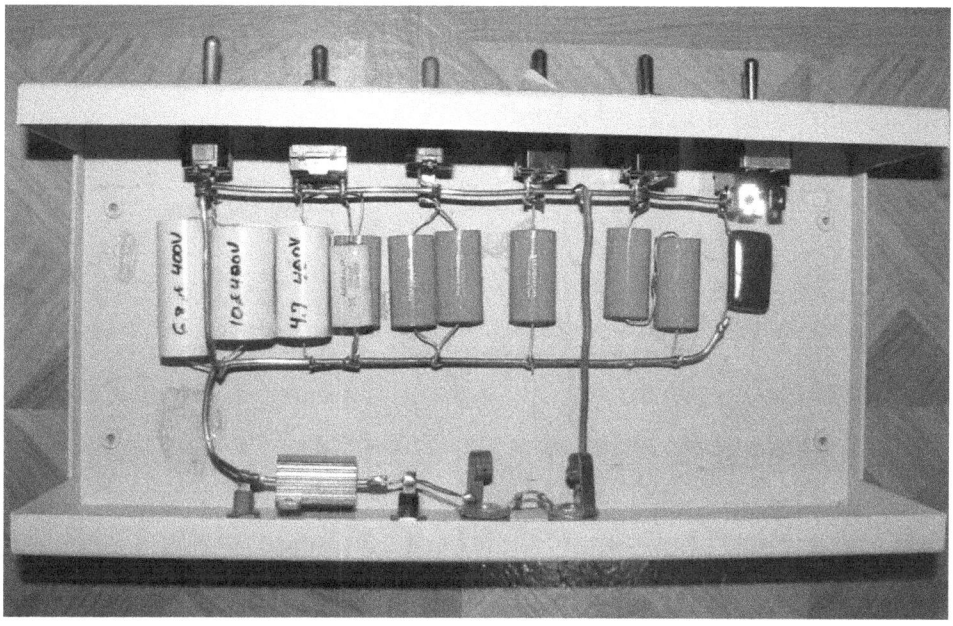

The signal generator can be a program that runs on your computer such as "Sweep generator". You can also use a frequency generator. Usually a sweep of several frequencies works best. For instance, a sweep might be from 600 to 620 cycles.

In the capacitor switch box, all of the capacitors must be arranged in parallel and or series to handle 400 volts minimum. Some of the capacitors "Doug" used were 2000 volt microwave oven capacitors. Although the audio amplifier is only putting out about 50 to 100 volts AC the coil/capacitor combination will kick back many times that voltage, typically 200 to 350 volts!

I sometimes use smaller coils that are made from 500 feet of 18 gauge magnet wire that measures 3.2 ohms. This is my favorite type of coil as it works with almost any amplifier. The bigger coils that are 500 feet of 12 or 14 gauge wire and measure 1.3 ohms, or less, will fry many an amplifier. My coils were wound on trash cans or on soda bottles. It turns out that coils made from 400 to 500 feet of wire are more effective than those made using 1000 feet. The longer lengths of wire increase the inductance and hence reduce the output current.

Basic Wire Size and Wire Length to Resistance;

Gauge AWG	Resistance per 500'	Resistance per 1000'	LBS Per 1000'
14	1.3	2.5	12
16	2.0	4.0	8
18	3.2	6.4	5
20	5.0	10.0	3

The above chart shows that 500 feet of 18 Gauge wire is 3.2 ohms, and that 500 feet of 20 Gauge wire is 5 ohms. A Coil of around 4 ohms is ideal for most "normal" audio amplifiers. So using 18 or 20 Gauge wire is the best choice for lots of power without overloading your coil driver or amplifier. If your amplifier can drive a two ohm load, like the QSC amplifier Doug used, then you could consider using 500 feet of 16 Gauge, or 14 Gauge wire.

If you are feeling risky you could even consider 500 feet of 12 Gauge wire, but that would overload and destroy almost any normal amplifier. That is why "Doug" used the QSC amplifier. The coil can also be made with enameled magnet wire, or with the larger gauge wires, thin insulation will also work. My favorite coil is 500 feet of 18 gauge wire.

The frequency generator can be a computer program or a frequency generator like the Heathkit Sine-Square Audio Generator Model IG-5218. I picked up a used one at a flea market for $25. It has knobs to select the frequency by dialing it in. However that model is not really "digital". It just uses some high precision resistors, so it can be off frequency by up to 5 cycles. I use my homemade frequency counter to keep the frequency fairly accurate. The Audio Generator replaced a program that I used to run on my Computer.

The square wave output of the frequency generator goes to the input of the audio power amplifier. I have used a Hafler PRO-5000 that is a 400 watt per channel audio amplifier as well as some QSC amplifiers. The amplifier output runs to the capacitor switchbox and then on to the coil. You can tell if it is working properly because the coil will get quite warm.

One way to wind a coil is to wind it on a plastic trash can. The taper of a trash can makes it easier to slide the completed coil off of the trash can. Once the coil is carefully removed, it then is wrapped in four evenly spaced places, with some electrical tape. Then the whole coil is wrapped in electrical tape. For a smaller coil, a one Gallon Ice Cream container works well. For an even smaller coil you can use a two liter soda bottle.

Basic Coil Setup;

      Frequency   Power
      Generator-------------Amplifier-------Capacitors-------Coil

When you are using the "Doug" coil setup it is important that the coil and the capacitors are tuned for the maximum output at any frequency. To do that, you can use an old CRT type of computer monitor or TV set. Then you can try capacitor values until you determine the settings needed to get the maximum output field strength as seen in the distortion that it causes on the screen. Switches can be marked 1, 2, 4, 8 and 16, for the uF of the capacitors. Using "Binary" you can then select values from 1 uF to 31 uF of capacitance by changing the switch settings. Never switch the capacitors while the amplifier is running at full power, always turn the power way down first. So far I have discovered that at 612 cycles per second, 8 uF is ideal for my favorite coil. Selecting the right value of capacitance will increase the magnetic field strength that is produced by as much as four times!

What are the Minimum Power Amplifier Requirements? How much power is needed to drive a 4 ohm coil? How about using as little as 120 watts! I have tried using a Sansui B-3000 audio amplifier driving a 4 ohm coil through the capacitor switch box. In the picture below you can see that the VU meter on the amplifier is completely pegged for this application. The amplifier protection circuit shuts off the amplifier if the input is too high, or if you try to drive it with a square wave.

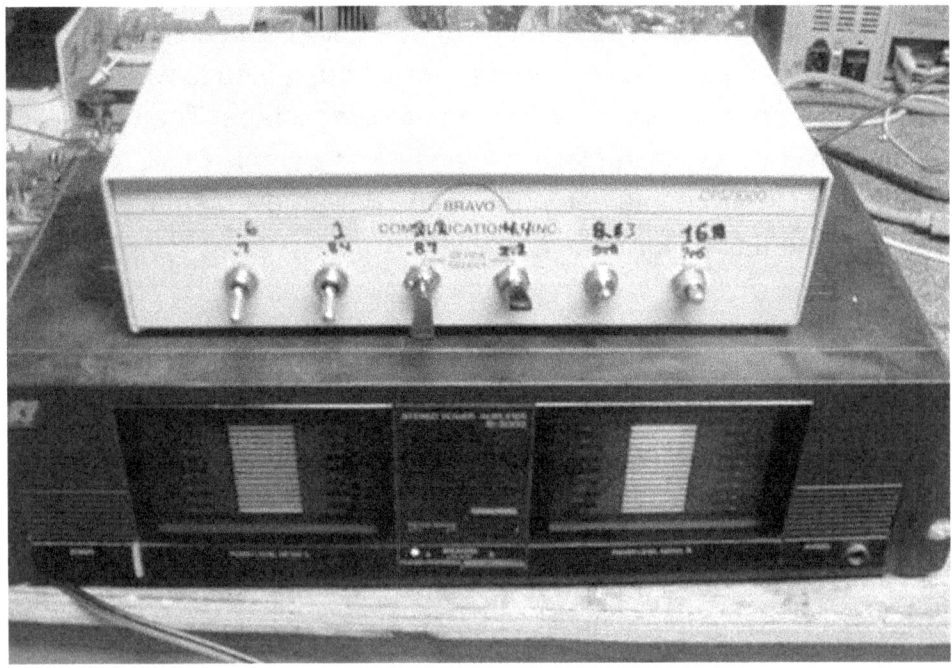

Using a QSC 1400 based Dough Coil Setup.

Another good amplifier to use for a low power Doug coil is the QSC 1400. It is rated at 200 watts per channel into eight ohms, and 300 watts per channel into four ohms. Like all QSC amplifiers it is very rugged and durable. I have rebuilt a few QSC 1400's myself and the only complaint is that they used older glass 3.9 volt zener diodes that have a high failure rate.

When the QSC 1400 is used to drive a four ohm coil, there was an output voltage of about 50 VAC. The volt meter showed about 170 VAC across the coil. The coil got hot very quickly. I was using 28 uF on the switch box for a 306 Hz frequency output. I have since added test points on the back of the capacitor box to make it easier to attach a voltmeter across the coil output.

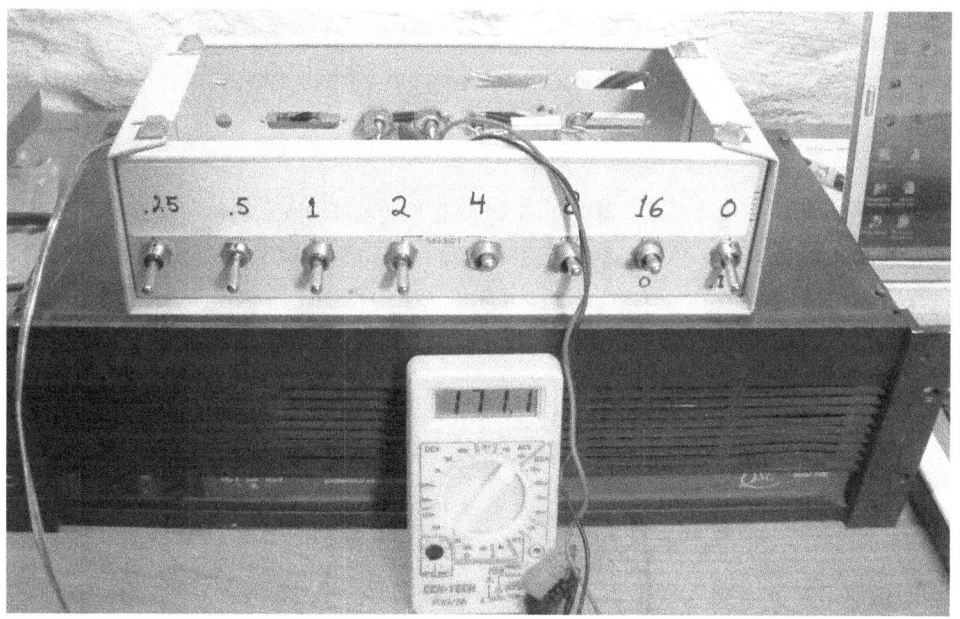

When I took the above picture the amplifier clipping light was blinking indicating that the amplifier was being driven almost to its maximum signal level.

Chapter 6

Alternate Coil Drivers,

Alternative Amplifiers

Years ago I set out to find or invent an alternate coil driver. First of all, there are cheaper amplifiers from QSC such as the USA 370 that can easily run a lower power version of the Doug Coil setup with a four ohm coil.

If you have some experience in building your own electronic circuits then you can save yourself some money on the cost of the high power amplifier. You can build your own home made coil driver circuit.

Eventually I came up with a two power FET coil driver design. It works in what is called class "D" as in "switching" mode, so it is much more power efficient than normal amplifiers.

Coming up on the next page there is a picture of the assembled project. What you see in the picture is two opto-couplers mounted on a small circuit board with the two power FET's visible in the background. Underneath the circuit board are the power supply filter capacitors.

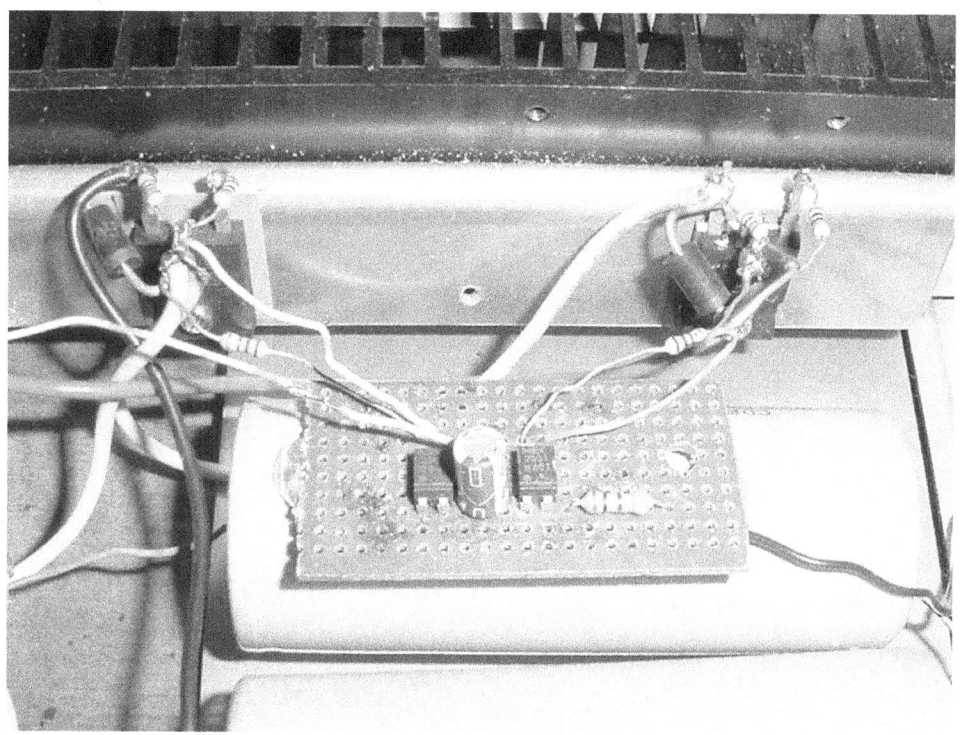

Coming up next is the FET coil Driver schematic diagram. Two opto-couplers handle all of the level switching and device driving functions. This use of opto-couplers greatly simplifies the driver design. It is sensitive enough to run off some computer headphone or speaker outputs.

In an earlier version there were two separate power supplies for the opto-couplers. Later on I figured out how to make one power supply run both the opto-couplers and the output power FET's.

Pulsed Electromagnetic Field Driver

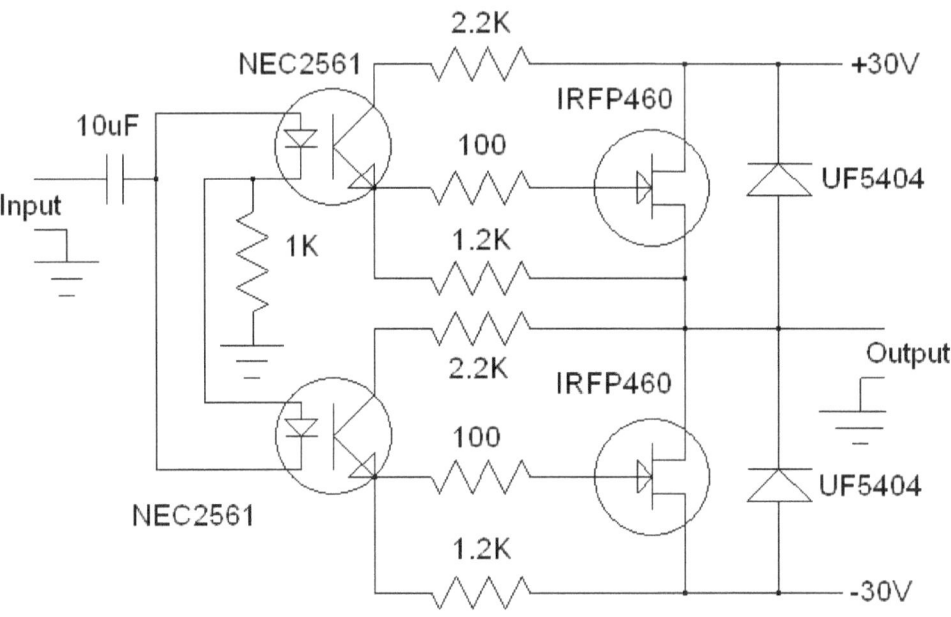

Below is a picture of what the output of this coil driver looks like on an oscilloscope screen. The square wave has some 60 cycle hum on it and the sine wave that comes from the coil is not a perfect sine wave, but the results are very similar what you get when you are using a sine wave to drive the coil.

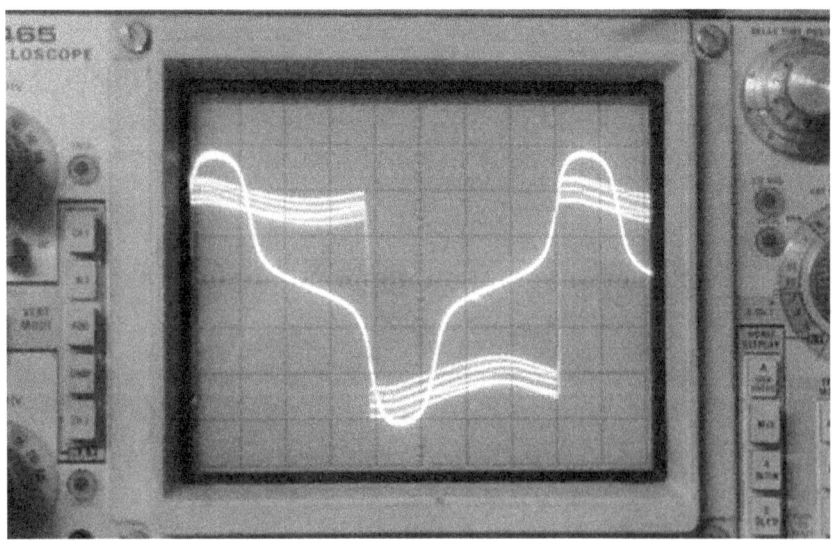

Here is a schematic of a typical power supply that can be used for this device as well as the next one. Do not forget to put a fuse or two in there.

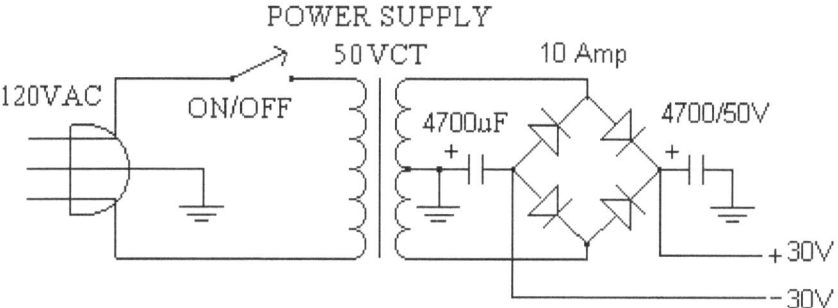

The L20 power amplifier design.

Another alternative coil driver that you can try is to buy an assembled and tested audio power amplifier circuit board on eBay. Below is a picture of one that is advertised on eBay as an "L20". It does not include the aluminum heat sink adapter that I have added. It is supposed to be able to deliver 350 watts RMS into 4 ohms. There are other models on eBay that are even more powerful.

For a power supply you will need a 50 to 60 volt center tapped power transformer capable of delivering about 8 amps. You will also need a bridge rectifier, and some filter capacitors to get it to work. Also, be sure to add some output fuses to protect the amplifier. There is a power supply transformer and rectifier circuit board for this amplifier that is also available on eBay.

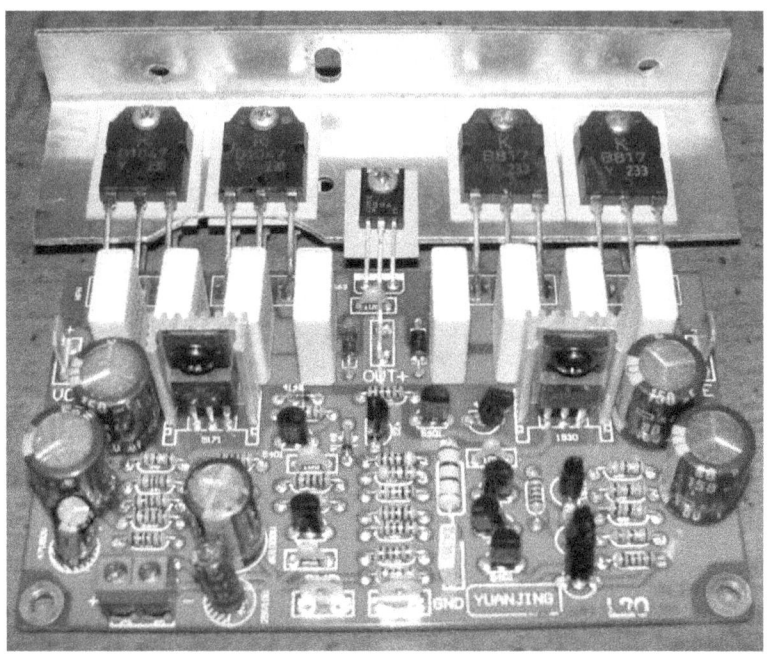

Coming up next is a picture of what it looks like installed inside of an amplifier. The positive wire is red, the negative wire is black and the speaker output is blue.

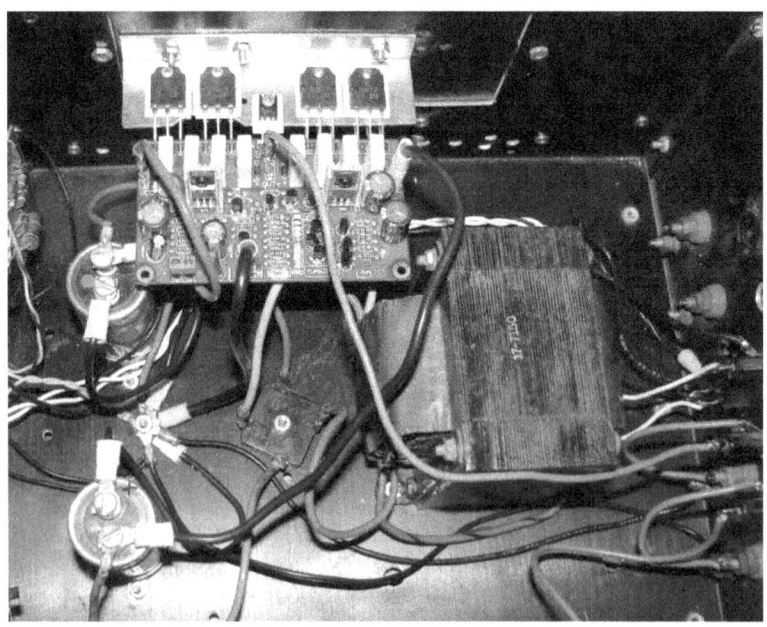

Chapter 7

Kirlian Photography,

Ozone Device

Kirlian photography takes picture of the tiny sparks that fly off the edges of things near a high voltage power supply. It claims to be able to detect diseases by where sparks are missing in the resulting picture. I personally do not think that claim is valid. However, using the Kirlian device does appear to help to treat some diseases.

This device works just like an ozone generator or an ozone based air purifier. An ozone generator uses two wavy metal plates, one on each side of a sheet of glass. High voltage is applied to the plates, and as air is blown through the waves in the metal, ozone is created and thrown off into the room.

In the Kirlian device, one of the metal plates is replaced with your hand. You can then see tiny sparks fly off your hand to the sheet of glass. Since you hand is now part of the ozone generator, ozone is being introduced directly into your blood stream. This reportedly treats open sores and some other conditions. It is thought that the ozone boosts your immune systems ability to fight anaerobic bacteria.

Below is a picture of the setup. Inside of the gray metal enclosure is a 12 volt power supply, a power transistor and a car ignition coil. The output of the coil goes through the green jumper wire to the copper plate that is below a sheet of glass that was removed from an old picture frame.

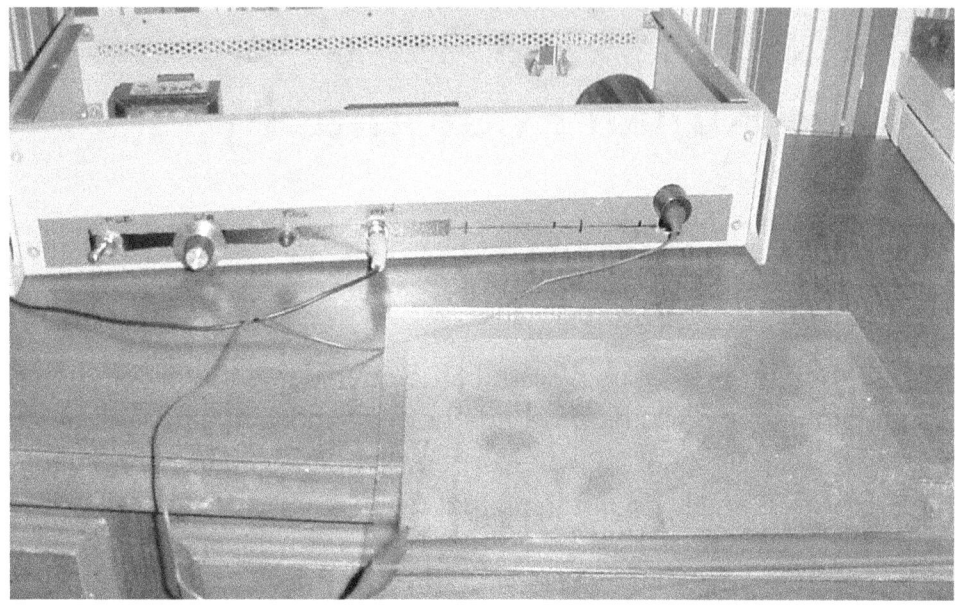

Coming up on the next page is the schematic diagram for a Kirlian type of device. A high power FET (Field Effect Transistor) works just as well as the 2N6057 power transistor if not better. The design difference with the FET the 1K resistor goes from the source to the ground. The signal generator can once again be a program running on your computer. Some computers will need an amplifier to get enough power to run this device. You can also use a signal generator as they have more power and generally work better.

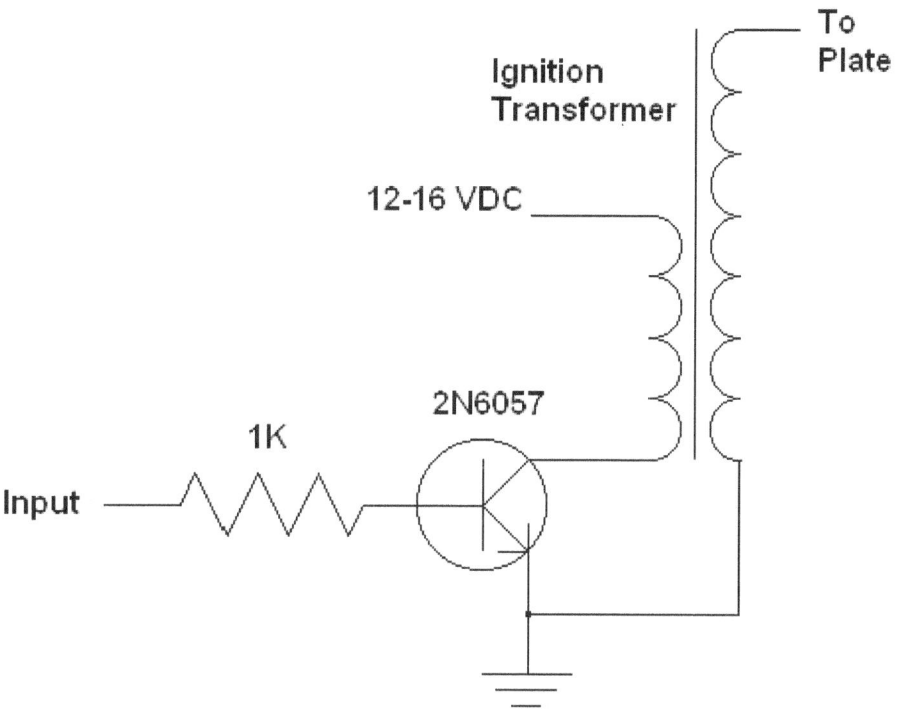

Here is a power supply to power the above circuit. The rectifiers should be rated for 4 Amps. The transformer is rated at 25VCT at 2 amps and is available at Radio Shack.

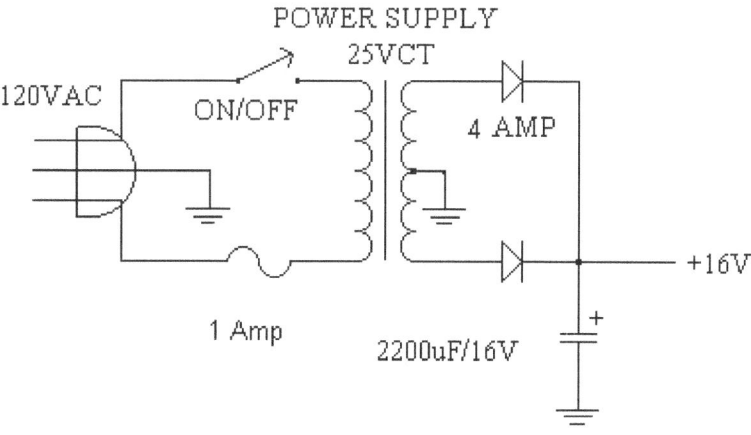

Chapter 8

Royal Rife,

Radio Frequency Transmitter

Rife reportedly cured about 16 people with terminal cancer using his device. It could even work when the equipment was located in a nearby room. It was even effective through the walls.

According to the story, he was given some terminal cancer patients that had failed all other attempts at treatment. He was able to cure about 12 of them with no problem. Then, after tuning up his equipment, he was able to cure the rest of them.

The Rife device is basically a vacuum tube powered AM radio transmitter. The modulation comes from an audio frequency generator. Most people think that Rife used an audio frequency that was around 2 KC to treat cancer. There are long lists of many other frequencies that were used to treat different conditions posted on the Internet.

Rife also invented a very complex special microscope, similar to what is now called a "Dark field microscope". With this special microscope he could see the germs and then he could determine what frequency would be the most effective at destroying the germs.

Here is a picture of a home made "Rife" device in operation. It used an 812 vacuum tube and a coil that was made to similar specifications to what some people have reported that Rife himself used.

The output tube that I used in this picture is a "U" shaped tube. This was all I had at that time, but it is not exactly what Rife himself used in his experiments. I hope to rebuild this Rife device on a metal chassis sometime in the near future.

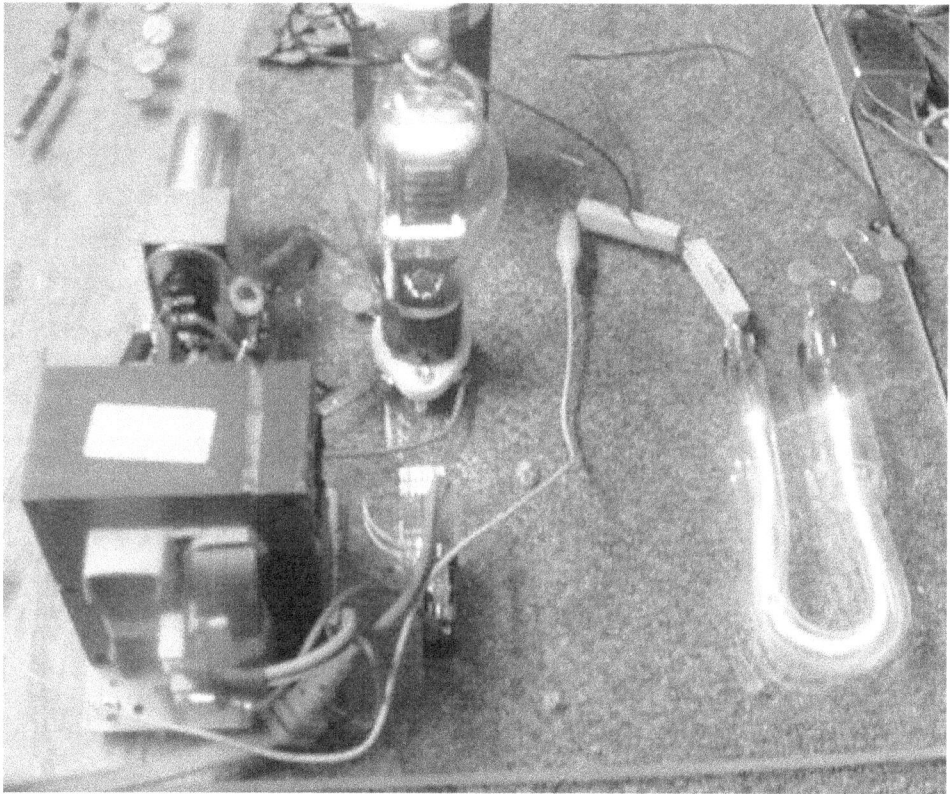

It took several tries to get my 812A vacuum tube Rife device to run without going up in smoke! Even though the schematic called for a 75 watt screen resistor, I tried a 10 watt resistor. I discovered that it would smoke after a few seconds of operation. The same applies to the ballast resistor. Currently I am using a 25 watt resistor for the screen resistor and two 10 watt resistors in series for the ballast resistor.

In the pictures you will see several capacitors in series. They are four .001 1KV capacitors in series to produce 250 PF at 4 KV as required by the schematic. Currently I do not have the 3000 volt insulated 10 Henry choke. There is lots of 60 cycles hum on the output signal as a result. Also the device that I made was not very stable in it's frequency of operation. It even caused interference with UHF reception on nearby TV's!

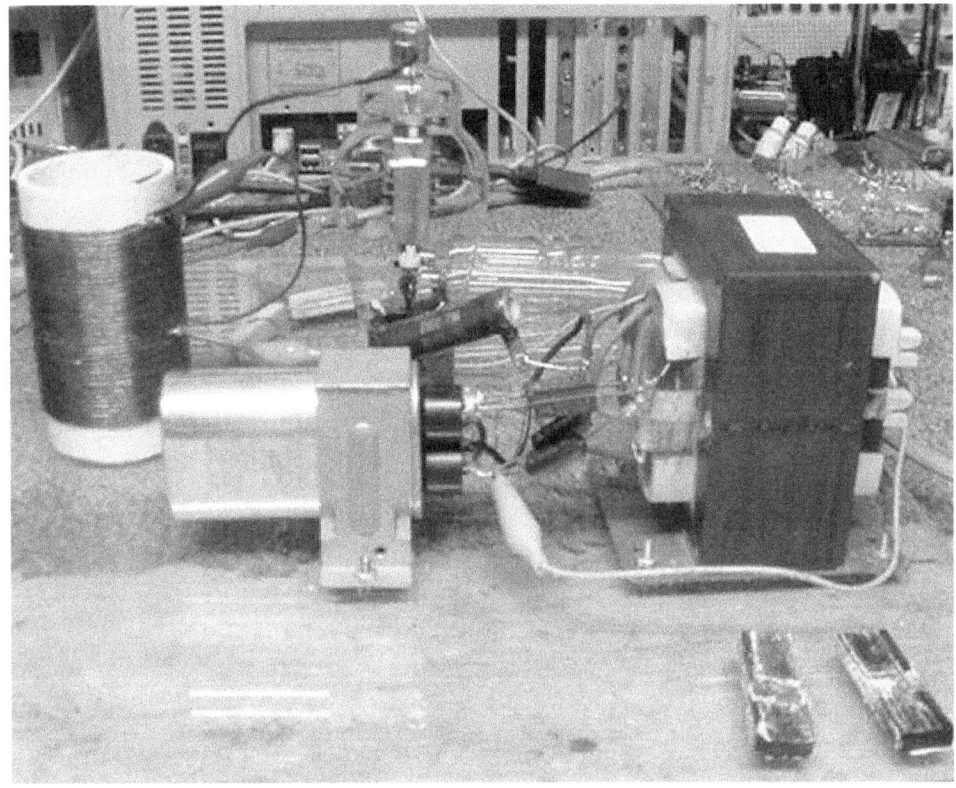

This picture show homemade parts that are needed to make it work. The first is the coil made from 40 turns of 16 gauge wire on a 2 1/2 inch form. It is tapped at turn 17. I used a piece of PVC pipe that is a little less than 2 1/2 inches in diameter. To space the wire, I used a smaller wire wound between the windings. Then I removed the smaller wire and covered the coil with glue. This technique works well with smaller gauge wire, but with this larger gauge wire the spacing did not hold very well.

For the power transformer I used a modified microwave oven transformer. First the two metal shims located between the windings have to be carefully removed. They are visible in the foreground of the above picture. Then I added four turns of 14 gauge THHN insulated wiring. This winding is then connected to the old, three volt filament winding, to get 6.5 volts for the 812 tube. From the looks of things 16 gauge wire would have done just as well.

Next I tapped the microwave oven transformer's high voltage winding about in the middle. It is impossible to find the exact center, so I used a bridge rectifier made out of four microwave oven diodes instead of the full wave rectifier that was shown in the schematic.

The ground wire that is located in the center of the transformer must be disconnected and insulated to use a bridge rectifier. Some schematics show only 600 volts on this power transformer.

First of all, I simplified the design from that of Rife's. The Rife schematic available elsewhere and on the Internet has the tap on the coil going to ground. It is simpler to have it go to the 1200 volt power source. The 2 uF capacitor is now 40 uF at 1600 volts, consisting of four 200 uF, 400V capacitors in series. This removes just about all the hum, without the need for a choke. There is a 10 Meg ohm resistor across them to discharge the high voltage, it takes several minutes.

You can use the primary winding of a 120 volt to 24 volt at 1/2 amp transformer for a choke coil if you still want one. The transformer will hum a lot when it is used as a choke coil. That is because it will be running on 120 cycles, not on the 60 cycles that it was designed for.

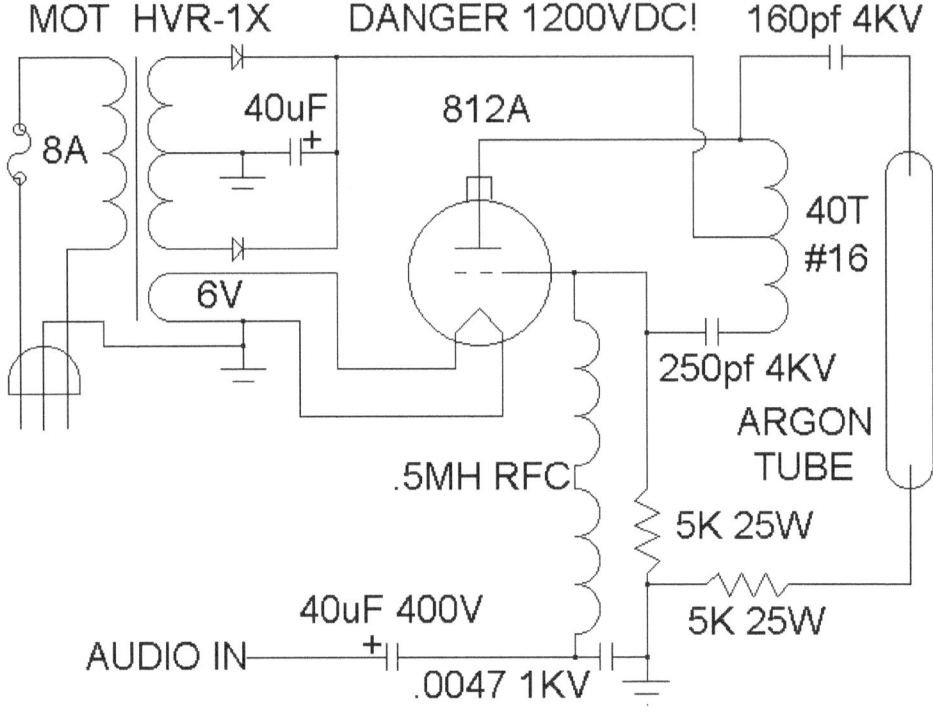

The 250 pF capacitor is made out of four .001 at 1 KV capacitors in series. The 160 pF capacitor is six .001 at 1 KV capacitors in series. The 5K resistors can be five 1K 10 watt resistors in series. My first attempts at modulating the signal resulted in the circuit breaker tripping. The choke had shorted out and was sending RF to ground. So I used two chokes to make sure that they would not short out again.

This next schematic is a schematic that is much closer to the original Rife design. In this schematic the coil tap at turn 17, is grounded instead of being connected to the power supply. This design requires a second high power RFC (Radio Frequency Choke) for the plate circuit of the 812 vacuum tube.

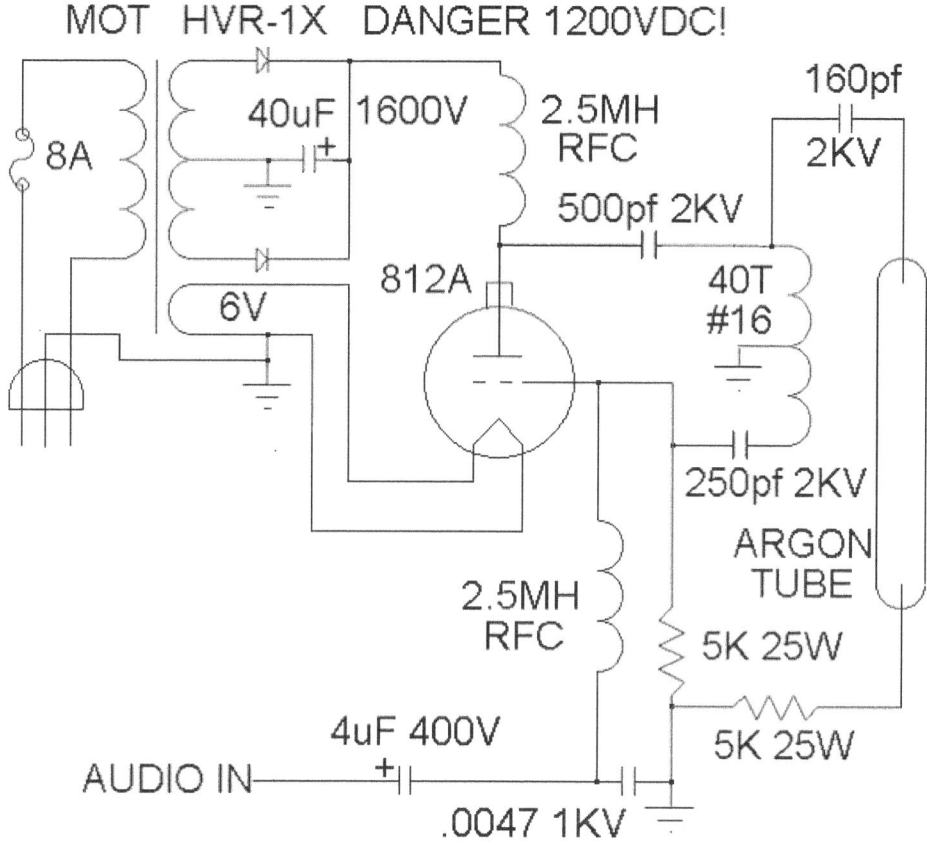

MOT HVR-1X DANGER 1200VDC!

Coming up next is the schematic of the audio driver circuit. This amplifier gives a gain of 22 and an output of up to 40 volts peak to peak to drive the audio input of the 812A Rife device. My signal generator has a maximum output of 10 volts peak to peak, but that is not enough to drive the vacuum tube. At first I was just using the two power transistors to go between the signal generator and the 812A Rife device. With that setup, there was only about 10% modulation.

When this Rife device was first fired up, the frequency counter went crazy and the signal was not modulated. It turns out that the audio signal needed more power to drive the 812 tube input. To give it more power, I added a 2N6050 transistor and a 2N6057 transistor as common emitter current boosters. At this point the signal is only modulated about 10% with the 10 Volts Peak to Peak from my signal generator.

So next I added the LF357 Op amp to give some more signal amplification. A 741 Op amp would likely work as well. Next the amplifier would also pick up a lot of RF noise so a .005 capacitor was added across the feedback resistor. A second .005 capacitor from the bases of the output transistors to ground may also be needed. The power supply for the Op amp should be regulated as most Op amps can not handle more than positive and negative 20 volts.

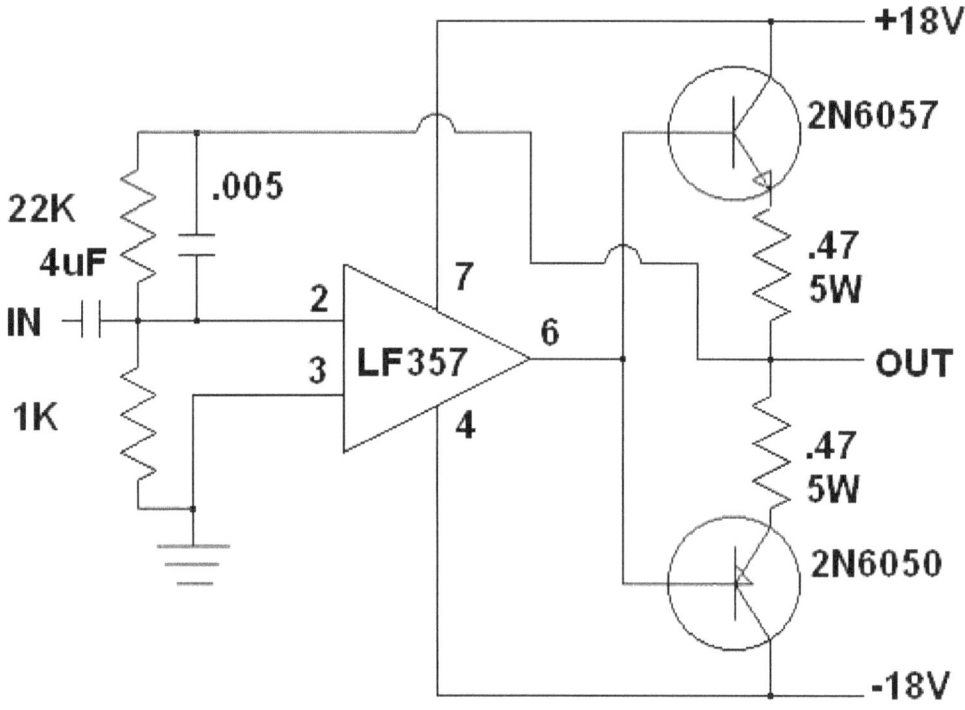

There is a more "modern" version of the Rife instrument that uses 27 MHz as the carrier frequency. That is the same frequency as CB radios use. Using that CB frequency makes the parts that are needed to build a Rife machine more readily available. Basically this setup uses an audio frequency generator feeding a CB radio. The output of the CB radio then goes to a 50 to 100 watt 27 Mz RF power amplifier. The output of the RF power amplifier then goes to the Rife tube.

The CB design is something that I have never tried. I also suspect that it would break a lot of the FCC regulations to broadcast that much power on the CB band. However there are a lot of CB addicts who broadcast at that much power all of the time and some how they get away with it.

Chapter 9

Poor Man's Rife,

Alternative Rife devices

Someone found a way to greatly simplify the Rife device and they developed what is usually referred to as a "Poor Man's Rife". This device usually uses a car spark plug coil to produce high voltage and a spark plug to create an arc. This arcing then becomes the carrier frequency for the Rife device.

My design is similar to the "Poor Mans Rife" but it uses an IRFP460 Power FET instead of a 2N6059 transistor. A 1K resistor goes from the gate (left terminal) to the ground (right terminal). The output of the FET is the middle terminal. The FET can handle 500 volts and 20 amps so it is much more powerful of a device than a transistor is.

The FET "ON" resistance is also much lower, so the FET runs very cool. As a result the high voltage from the ignition coil is MUCH higher than when using a transistor. It will jump a 1/8 inch gap and still have lots of power to light the argon tube. The spark gap is any spark plug.

An optional capacitor across the coil primary is a .047 at 600 volt device. I left out that capacitor out of some of my schematics. What that capacitor does is reduce the rise and fall times and increase the output by about 10% to 20%. The 1 K ohm resistor is also optional, it protects the FET from static and prevents it from conducting when there is no input signal. The Power FET should be mounted on a heat sink such as a piece of aluminum.

Below is a picture of a "Poor Man's Rife" machine in operation. In the picture, the vacuum tube that is used to transmit the resulting signal has a large bulge in the center. This is the type of tube that Royal Rife himself used. It has 2 plates inside of it, one on a 45 degree angle. The vacuum tube is filled with a gas such as argon. The program Sweep Generator is running on my laptop computer.

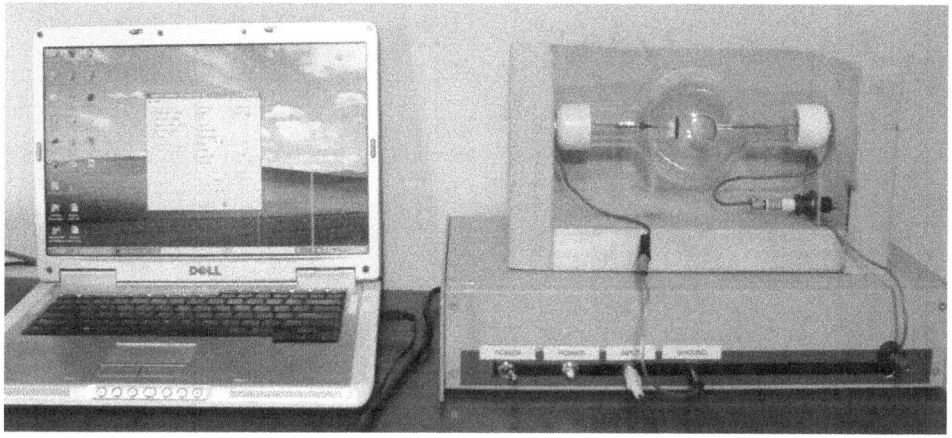

The next picture is a close up of the output tube while it is running, the color on one plate is blue, but the color on the other plate is purple.

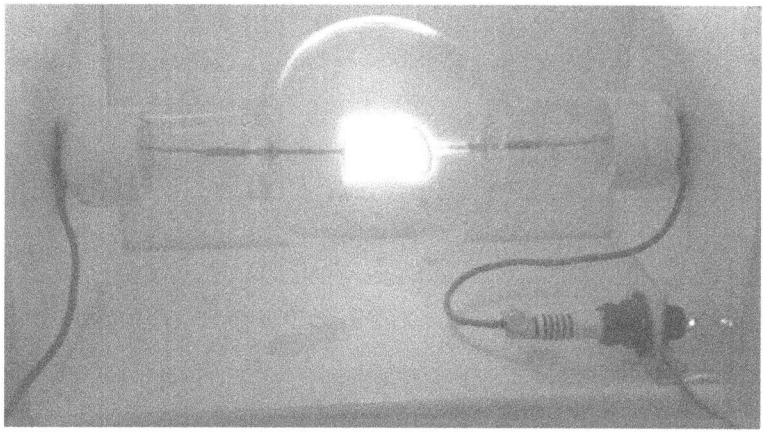

Here is the schematic of my poor man's Rife machine. The spark plug is drawn as two dots in the upper right corner in the schematic; it goes between the high voltage output of the coil and the argon tube. It runs on 16 Volts at 4 Amps, although the schematic says 12V.

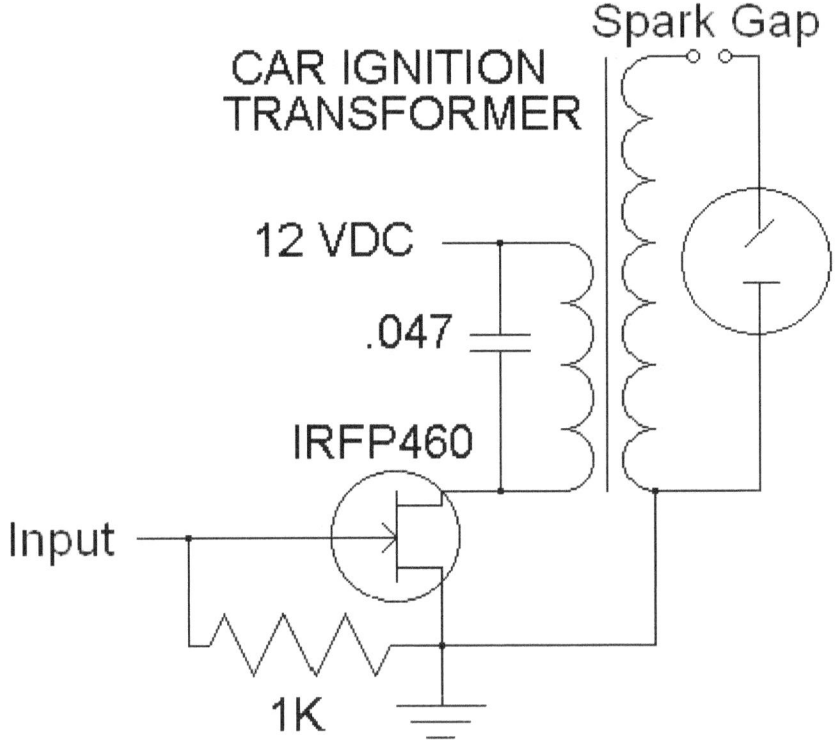

The next picture is what the power supply looks like, inside of the cabinet. The 25VCT 2 amp power transformer is on the left. Below that is a 741 audio amplifier that is needed to work with some computer outputs. The big heat sink in the center holds the power FET. On the right is a used car spark plug coil. A strap of 12 gauge wire was added to hold the coil in place.

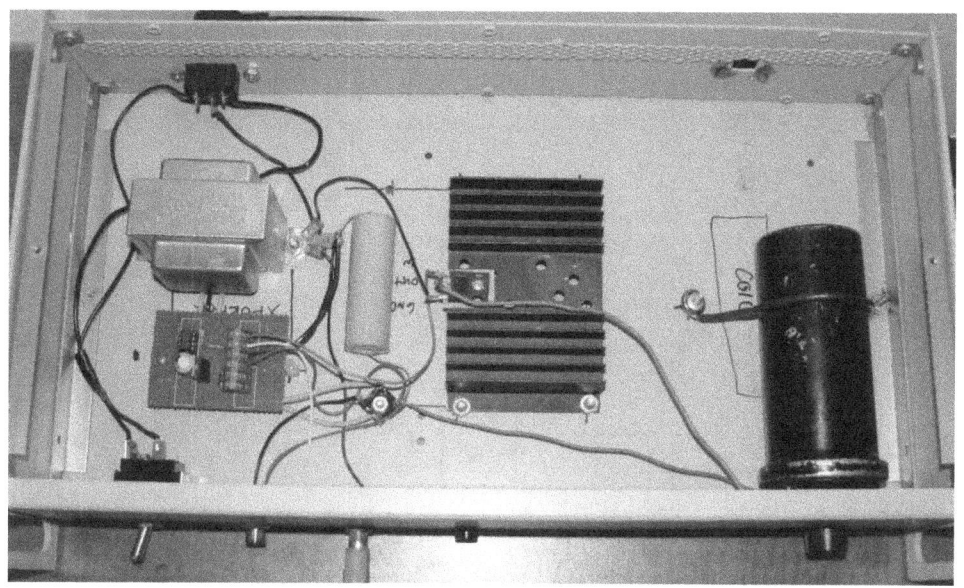

Next there is the schematic diagram of the optional audio buffer amplifier for use with some computer outputs that do not have enough power to drive this device. This buffer amplifier would likely work with other devices in this book that do not work with some computer outputs that are too low to drive them.

The buffer amplifier has a gain of about seven, so a one volt input signal gives you a seven volt output signal. If that is not enough gain you can change the 15 K ohm resistor to 10 K ohm instead for a gain of about 10x.

BUFFER AMPLIFIER

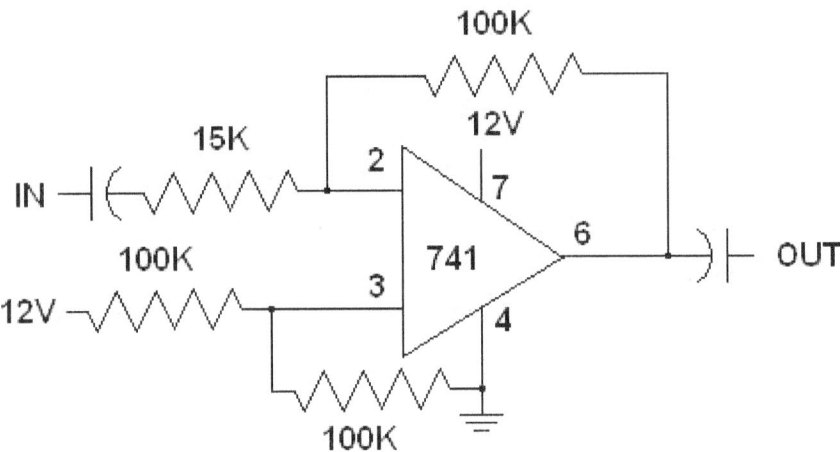

Next up is the schematic of the power supply. Be aware that the 25 VCT 2 amp power transformer from Radio Shack gets very hot. A bigger transformer might work a little better. The 12 volt output is for the buffer amplifier and it has a 100 uF at 16 volt capacitor to ground on its output. The 16 volt output goes to the car ignition coil.

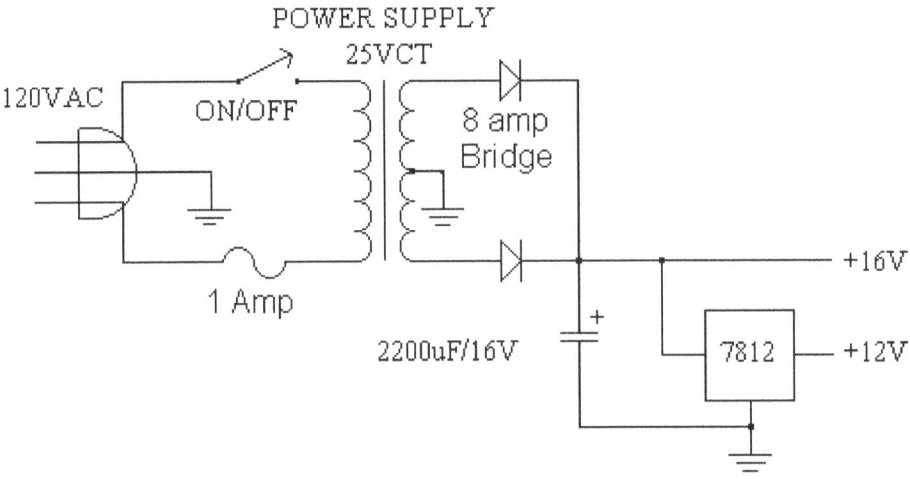

Parts list for poor mans Rife machine:
1 – 25 VCT 2 amp power transformer
1 – 8 amp bridge rectifier
1 – 2200 at 25 volt capacitor

1 – Power switch
1 – Power jack
1 – 1 Amp fuse and holder
1 – 1 K ohm 1/2 watt resistor
1 – IRFP460 FET capable of 20 Amps
1 - .047 250 volt paper capacitor
1 – Older Car ignition transformer

Parts list for optional amplifier
1 – LM7812 voltage regulator
1 – 100 uF at 16 volts
1 – 741 op amp and IC socket
3 – 100 K 1/4 watt resistors
1 – 15 K 1/4 watt resistor
2 – 10 uF at 25 V capacitors

Chapter 10

Making Your Own Colloidal Silver

Colloidal silver can be made in a glass with two five or six inch 12 to 18 gauge silver rods, two jumper wires, distilled water, and two or three nine volt batteries. The batteries can be used ones from smoke detectors, etc. Rinse out a class or canning jar with the distilled water, and then fill it with the distilled water. Bend a one half inch U in one end of each of the silver rods and insert them in the distilled water on opposite sides so that they do not touch each other. Connect the batteries two hours you should have some colloidal silver. It is best to put a plastic cover over the jar to keep dust out.

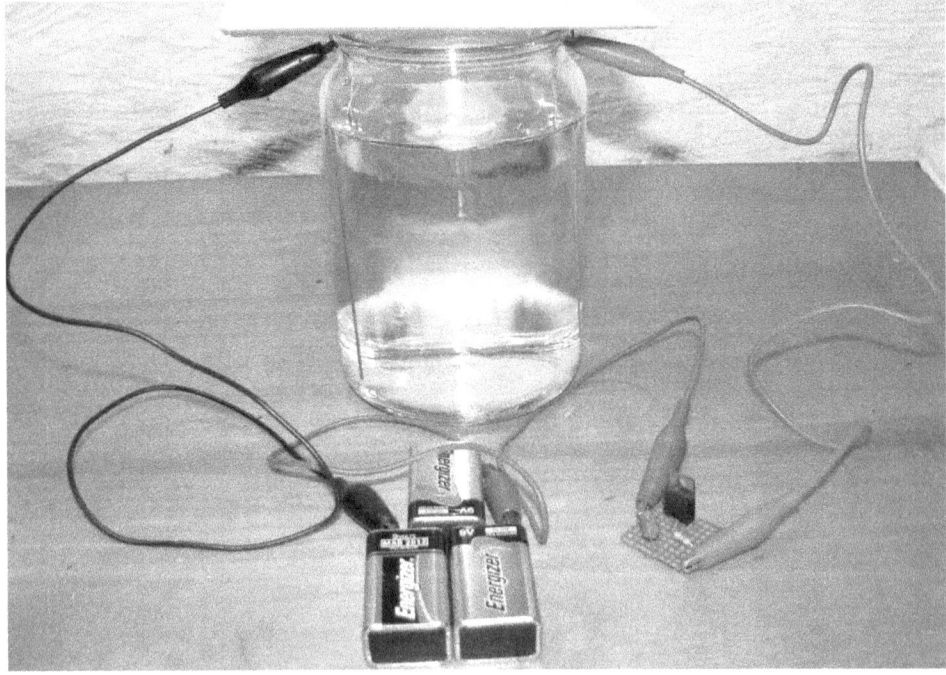

There are several complications to making your own colloidal silver. The first and biggest problem is current runaway that will "burn" the silver resulting in large grey chunks. The burnt chunks can be filtered out with a coffee maker filter, but it is much better not to make any to start with. There are several solutions to use to prevent the burning of the silver. The first solution is to stir the water periodically so the silver ions do not all concentrate in the center between the rods. Stirring can be manually done every five minutes, or it can be automated.

There are three ways to automatically stirring the distilled water. One method is to use a fish tank air bubbler. The drawback of the air bubbler method is that you might be putting dust from the air into your colloidal silver solution. A second device to use is called a magnetic stirrer. You put a magnet in the bottom of the jar and apply an AC field under the jar to make the magnet spin and hence stir the liquid.

Another automatic stirring method is to mount a small incandescent light bulb a few inches underneath the water container. The heat from the light bulb will cause the water to circulate. It will also speed up the electrolysis process so the colloidal silver can be produced faster at higher concentrations.

Another way to help prevent current runaway is to add a current limiter circuit. You can make a current limiter from a voltage regulator IC with the wiring configuration changed to make it into a current regulator instead. Most people use a LM7805 as the current regulator because it is the most common regulator, but a LM7812 regulator would also work if the resistor value was changed. We want to limit the current to between two and ten milliamp (that is .010 amps) maximum to produce the smallest particles of silver.

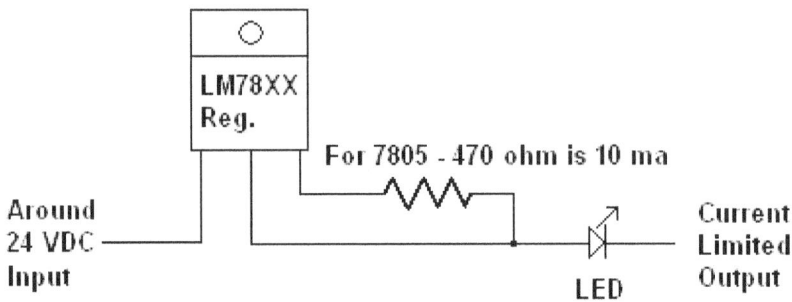

For 7805 - 470 ohm is 10 ma

Around
24 VDC
Input

Current
Limited
Output

LED

Output Current = (Output Voltage) / R

Here is a picture of the current regulator.

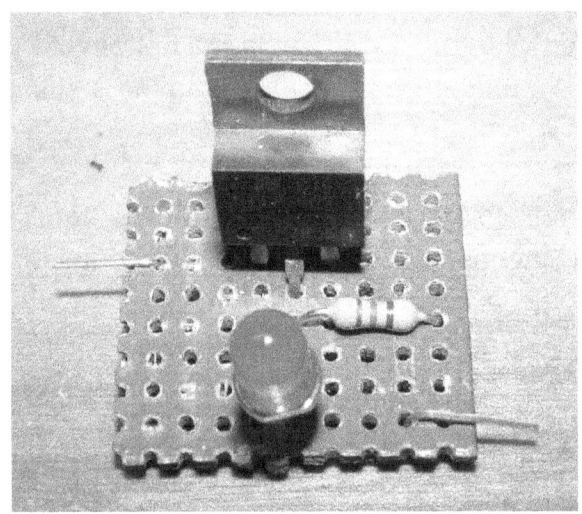

Another problem with making your own colloidal silver is that one of the silver rods will be coated with crud. One solution to this problem is to periodically clean the silver rod with a clean paper towel. Another solution is to reverse the power polarity manually or automatically. A 555 timer and a relay can be used to automatically reverse the polarity and keep the silver rods clean.

A final device to use is a timer. If you forget about the silver maker, the silver can get burnt. So any kitchen timer can be used to remind yourself to check on the silver or an electronic timer can turn off the silver maker off automatically.

Do not even think about using tap water, the chlorine in it is deadly. I discovered this years ago. I was carrying water from the house to water my garden, but the garden was doing terrible. Someone told me to use pond water instead. Sure enough when I started using pond water the garden really took off. I have seen this demonstrated time and time again. If you do not have a pond or creek, use a 5 gallon pail to collect rain water from your eves. But remember this: If tap water kills your plants, imagine what it is doing to you.

Also do not add salt or anything other than heat to make the colloidal silver generator work faster. Any chemical you use will mess with the silver and can produce toxic byproducts.

Chapter 11

Arduino Controlled

Colloidal Silver Maker

I have used a colloidal silver maker for years, but it was not mine, and the owner asked for it back. Then I looked for my home made colloidal silver maker but could not find it. I have way too much junk to look through. Then I got an idea, why not make a colloidal silver maker that is powered by an Arduino so it could control the voltage, current, reverse the polarity, record the results and even time the operation.

This is my latest schematic of the interface to the colloidal silver maker. I used a L293 motor controller because it supports reversing the polarity and can easily run the stirrer motor.

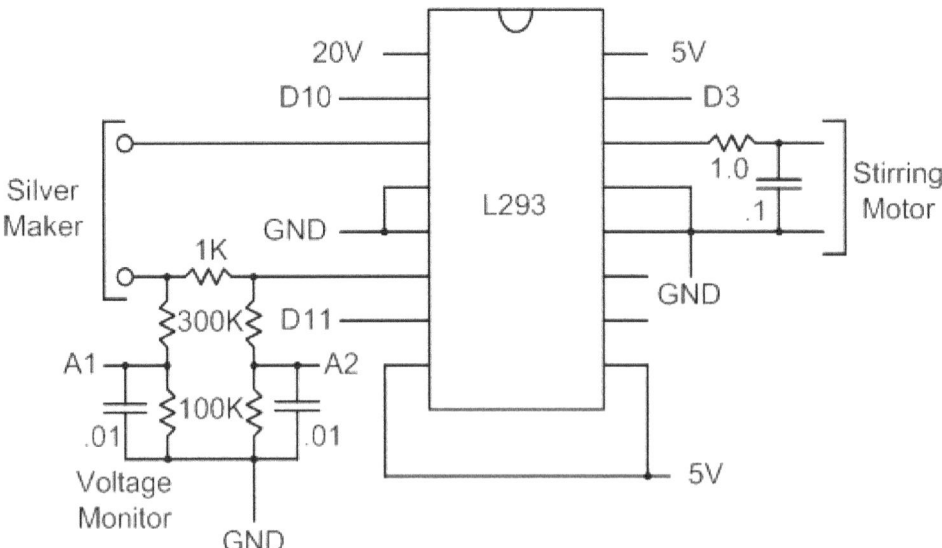

I had to add some filter capacitors in the circuit to attempt to get more stable numbers for the LCD display and to prevent premature shut off. I have changed the resistors in the divider to 300K (Two 150K in series) and 100K to further reduce the current reading when there is no water is present. Also note that the stirrer motor is now on D3 for PWM speed control ability. Eventually you might be able to adjust the stirrer motors voltage with a few key presses. I have also made a small circuit board with the voltage and current monitoring resistors on it. This circuit board is visible in some of the latest pictures.

This is the schematic diagram showing the 1602 LCD wiring. This is identical to the LCD shield wiring commonly available on eBay.

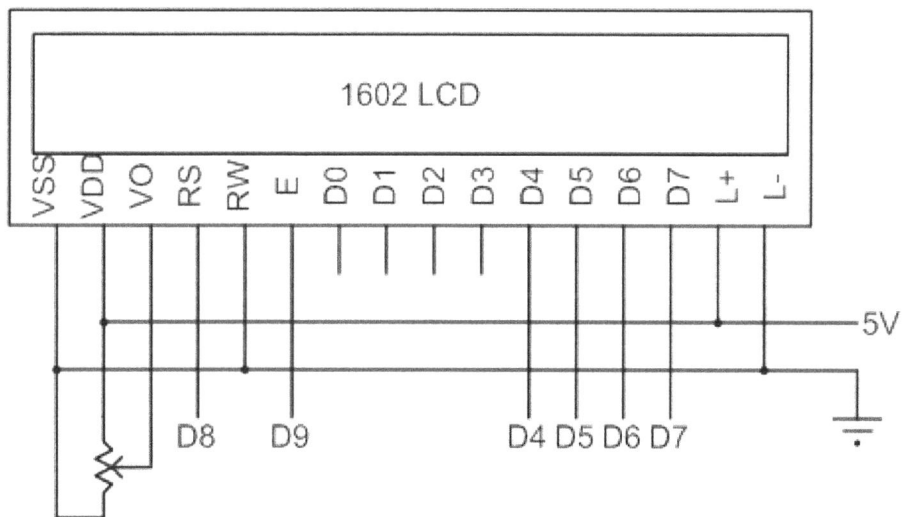

This is what the LCD screen looks like in an earlier version. I could use a bigger screen! The LCD is saying the voltage is .51 volts and .25 volts across a 1K ohm resistor for a current of .25ma; it usually never reaches 1 ma during over 4 hours of operation. Every 30 minutes the Arduino reverses the polarity and the LCD will then show around 17.7 volts. The bottom line of the LCD also displays the run time.

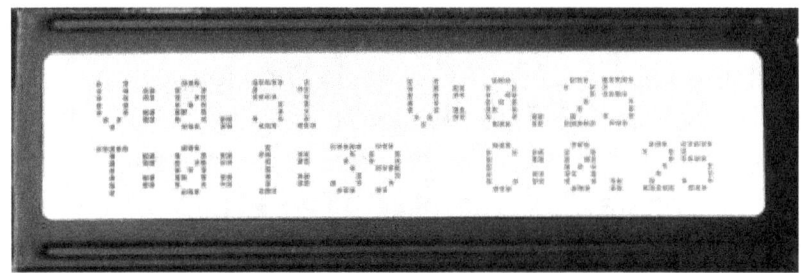

This is what the LCD looks like after over 30 minutes of operation, when the polarity has been reversed. The voltage and current bounce around a lot, likely because of the noise from the air pump motor.

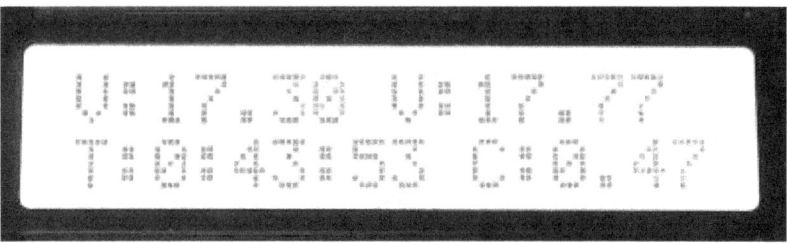

Up next is a picture of the colloidal silver maker, when it was still using a breadboard. The L293 motor control board is visible on the right side of the picture. This picture shows the Colloidal Silver Generator actually running. The Air pump stirrer has been added with 20 ohms in series to reduce the motor noise. Also the motor ground must be separate from the other grounds because of all the electrical noise that the motor makes.

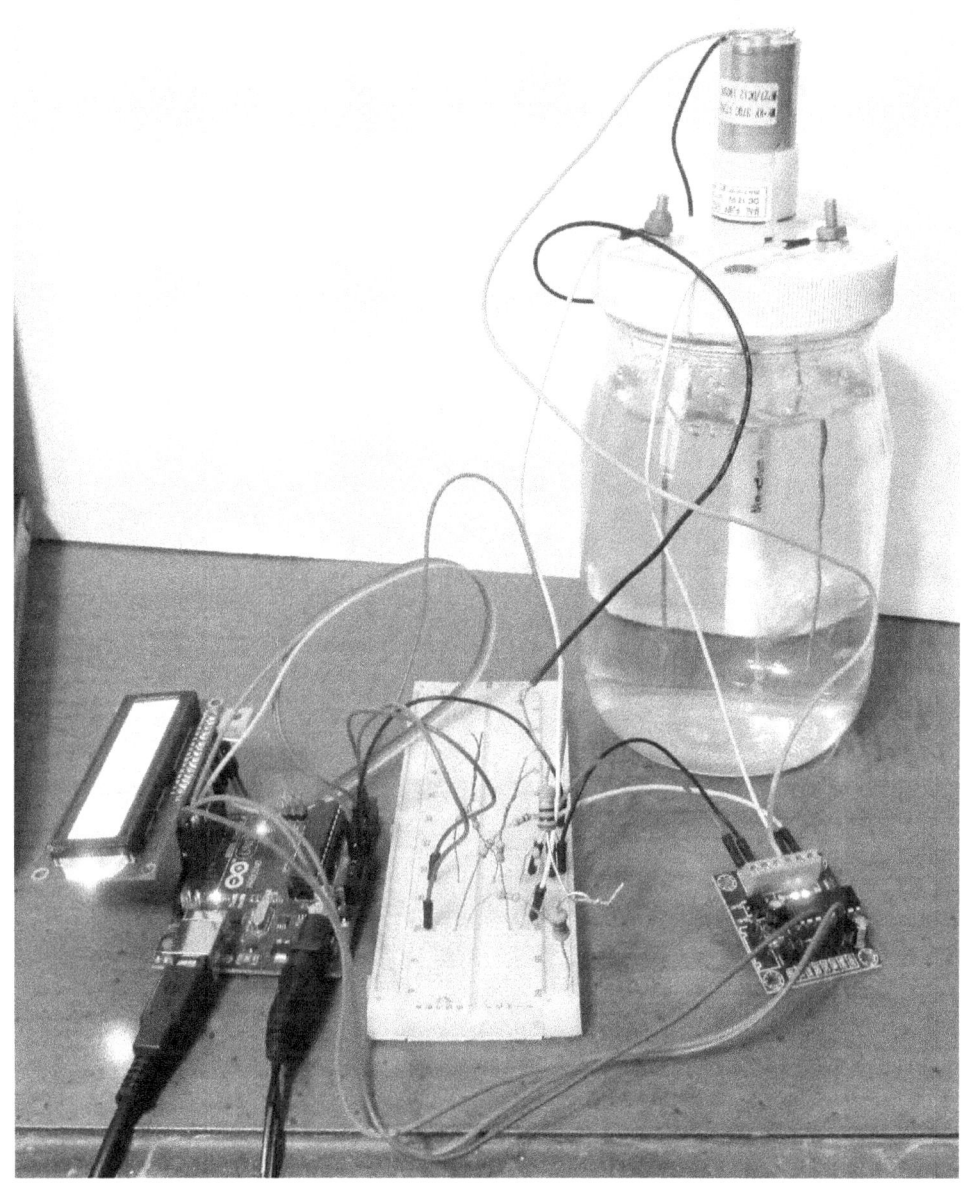

Here is another picture, this time it is the completed colloidal silver maker. The resistor divider and L293 motor controller are now located on the top of the colloidal silver maker. Eight wires then run down to the Arduino. There are two ground wires, one ground wire for the motor controller and one ground wire for the voltage divider.

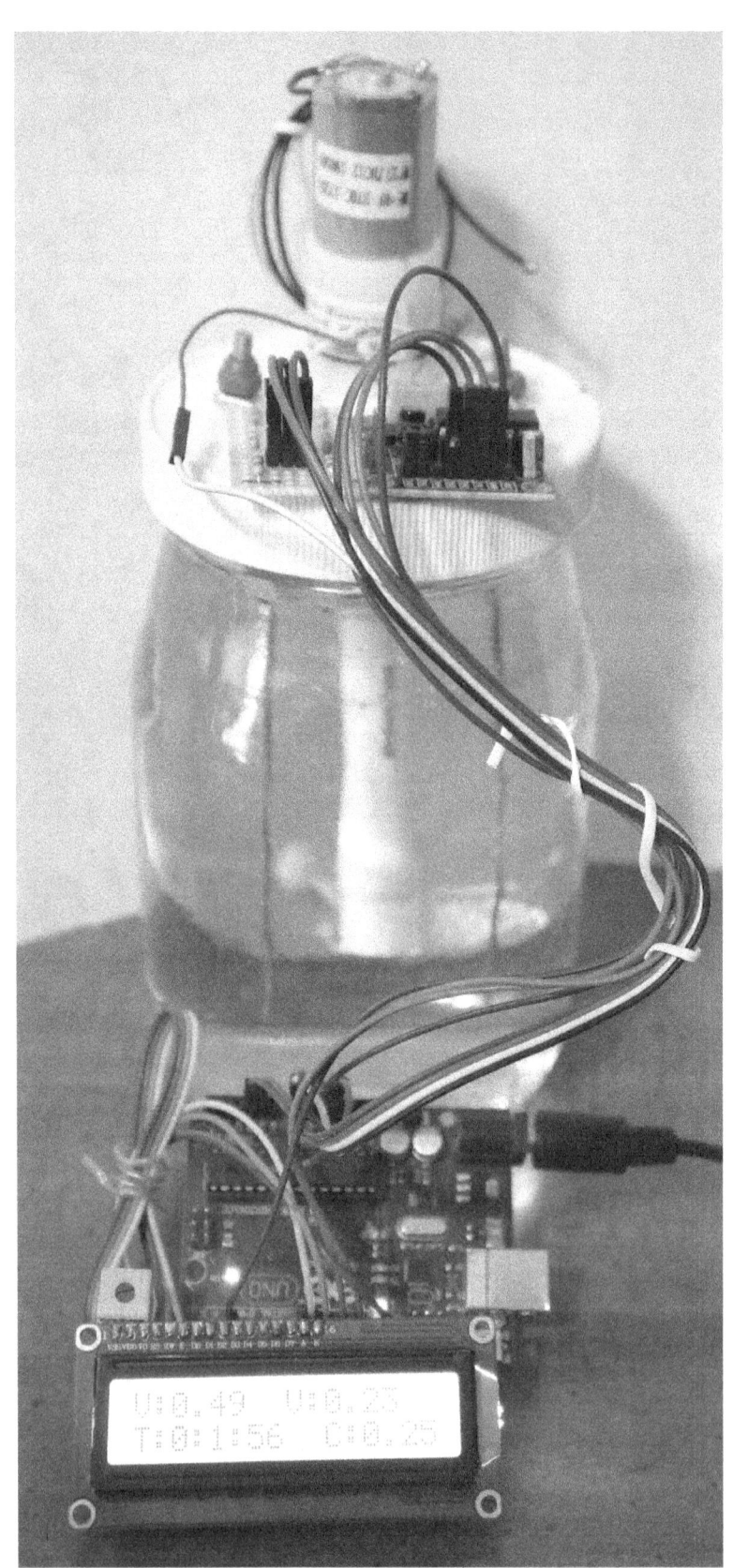

After the second test run with the current staying under .5 ma, and 1 ma being the ideal current, I am thinking that it needs to to be modified from 12 volts to 20 volt operation. Most Colloidal silver makers use 24 to 28 volts. The L293 can operate up to 30 volts, but the Arduino voltage regulator has a maximum of 20 volts, and the air pump stirrer has a maximum of 12 volts. The air pump runs best at around 9 volts. So either a redesign will be needed to have some voltage regulators added, or I can try to use a 20 volt power source like that of an old laptop ac adapter.

I tested this design for a few minutes with a 19 volt laptop AC adapter. Only 17.7 volts made it to the colloidal silver maker. The Arduino voltage regulator got very warm but survived. I disconnected the air pump for this test because it is rated for 12 volts maximum and runs best at 7-9 volts. I have since added a PWM output from the Arduino for the air pump of 1/2 of the power source or 10 volts for 20 volt operation.

The Arduino's PWM ability is used to regulate the current to the Colloidal Silver maker to just under 1 ma. The over-current shutdown is set to 2.0 ma.

Here is the code so far:

```
/***************************
Arduino Colloidal Silver Maker
By Bob Davis
April 2020

Use a 16x2 LCD display shield or equivalent
Shows the voltage, current, and run time.

The circuit:
 * LCD RS - D9
 * LCD Enable - D8
 * LCD D4 - D4
 * LCD D5 - D5
 * LCD D6 - D6
```

* LCD D7 - D7
* LCD R/W and VSS pin to ground
* LCD VCC and LED pin to 5V
* 10K variable resistor:
* ends to +5V and ground
* wiper to LCD VO pin (pin 3)
* Uses L293 motor controller on D10 and D11 for PWM ability
* Uses L293 on D3 for stirrer motor.

*********************/

```
// include the library code:
#include <LiquidCrystal.h>

// initialize the library with the numbers of the

interface pins
LiquidCrystal lcd(9, 8, 4, 5, 6, 7);

// Pins for Colloidal silver maker
int CS1=10;
int CS2=11;
// Pins for stirrer
int Stir=3;
int Shutdown=0;
// Variables for time
int hours;
int minutes;
int seconds;
long hour = 3600000; // 3600000 milliseconds in an hour
long minute = 60000; // 60000 milliseconds in a minute
long second = 1000; // 1000 milliseconds in a second
float AN1=0.0; // Analog input 1
float AN2=0.0;
float temp1=0.0;
float temp2=0.0;
float CUR=0.0;  // Current in ma
int CurSet=255; // Current Setting

void setup() {
  // set up the LCD's number of columns and rows:
```

```
  lcd.begin(16, 2);
  pinMode (CS1, OUTPUT);
  pinMode (CS2, OUTPUT);
  pinMode (Stir, OUTPUT);
}

void loop() {
  // Reverse current every 30 minutes
  if (Shutdown==0){
    analogWrite(Stir, 128); // 1/2 supply voltage
    if (minutes<30){
      analogWrite(CS1, 0);
      analogWrite(CS2, CurSet);
    }
    else{
      analogWrite(CS2, 0);
      analogWrite(CS1, CurSet);
    }
  }
  else{
    analogWrite(CS1, 0);
    analogWrite(CS2, 0);
    analogWrite(Stir, 0);
    }
  temp1=analogRead(A1);
  AN1=((temp1*5.0)/1024.0)*4.0;
  temp2=analogRead(A2);
  AN2=((temp2*5.0)/1024.0)*4.0;
  CUR=abs(AN1-AN2);
  if (CUR > 1.0) {CurSet--;} // Reduce PWM
  lcd.clear();
  lcd.setCursor(0,0);
  lcd.print("V:");
  lcd.print(AN1);
  lcd.setCursor(8,0);
  lcd.print("V:");
  lcd.print(AN2);
  lcd.setCursor(10,1);
  lcd.print("C:");
  lcd.print(CUR);
  // print the number of seconds since reset:
```

```
long timeNow = millis();
hours = (timeNow) / hour;
minutes = ((timeNow) % hour) / minute ;
seconds = (((timeNow) % hour) % minute) / second;
lcd.setCursor(0, 1);
lcd.print("T:");
lcd.print(hours);
lcd.print(":");
lcd.print(minutes);
lcd.print(":");
lcd.print(seconds);

if (hours>3){ // Time under 4 hours
  Shutdown=1;
  }
if (CUR>2.0){ // Current under 1ma
  Shutdown=1;
  }

delay(300);
}
```

Chapter 12

Signal Generators

We are going to look at three types of signal generators. There is SweepGen a software based signal generator that requires a computer. Next there is a DDS signal generator that generates a fixed frequency. Last of all there is a DDS sweeping signal generator that can produce a range of frequencies.

SweepGen can be run as a fixed frequency generator or as a sweep generator. Here is a picture showing both setups. On the left there is "No sweep" selected and a fixed frequency of 306 hertz. You need to manually type in the frequency. On the right there is a slow sweep from 300 to 330 hertz.

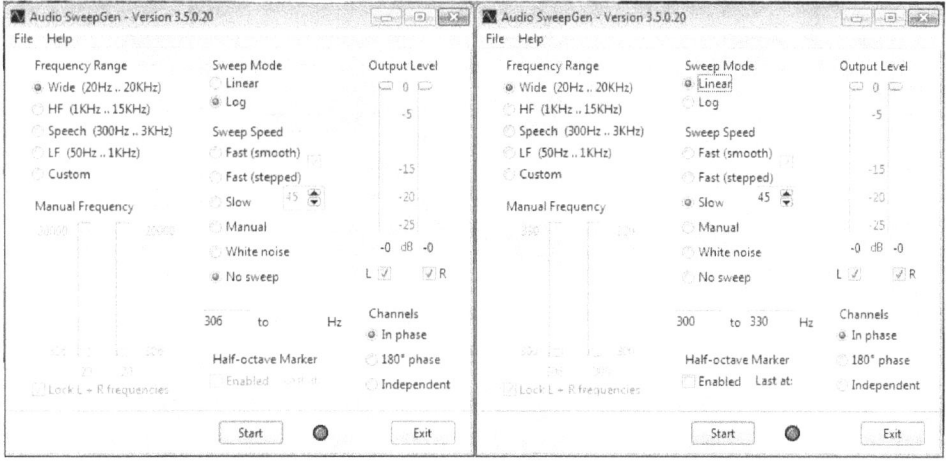

Most computers do not have a lot of output signal voltage. As you can see the volume controls are turned all the way up. The speaker on the task bar also needs to be turned all the way up.

"DDS" Stands for "Direct Digital Synthesis". I recently purchased a function/signal generator on eBay. This was purchased for two reasons. My computer based signal generator was limited to a top frequency of only 20 KHz and I wanted one that would go a little higher. Secondly I also wanted a signal generator for inclusion in this book. This signal generator was included for people who do not have, or do not know how to use, a computer based frequency generator. I was delighted that this signal generator works great, and that the very limited instructions that came with it do in fact cover what is needed to get it to work.

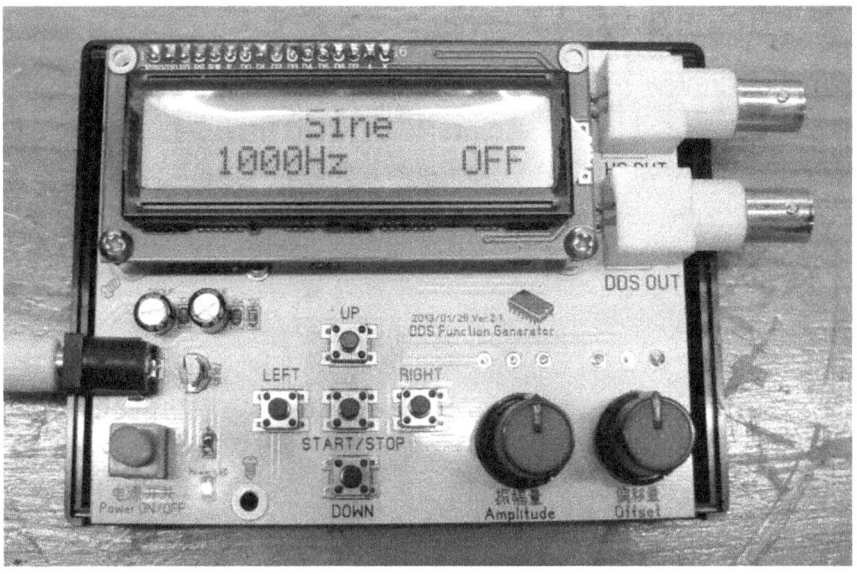

I added spacers under the bottom two corners of the LCD to hold it in place and hot melt glued the function generator into a 3.25 inch by 4.25 inch project box. I had to trim the bottom edge of the project box as the circuit board was just a little bit too big to fit otherwise. A box that was 4 inches by 3.25 inches would have been a better fit.

My function generator did not come with a back-lit LCD so I swapped another LCD in. It is a standard 1602 LCD display. At first it did not work at all! There were two problems with the change.

The first problem is a 50 ohm resistor above the LCD jack that needs to be soldered in for the back-light. On models without a back light the resistor is left out.

The second problem is that the LCD contrast trimmer is located underneath the LCD. You have to play with it to get the right setting. I was tempted to unsolder the trimmer resistor's single or center pin. Then bend the variable resistor up on the other two pins and then solder a jumper from the single pin to the circuit board. That way you could adjust the trimmer while watching the LCD to see if what is the best setting.

The function generator will run on a 9V AC adapter or on a 9 volt battery with no problems. What the signal generator is equivalent to is an Arduino with a resistor ladder based analog to digital converter on several output pins. Then there is an Op amp buffer amplifier to drive the output jacks.

I was able to find this schematic diagram located on the next page. It is of an earlier version of the device. Sorry if the schematic is not very clear.

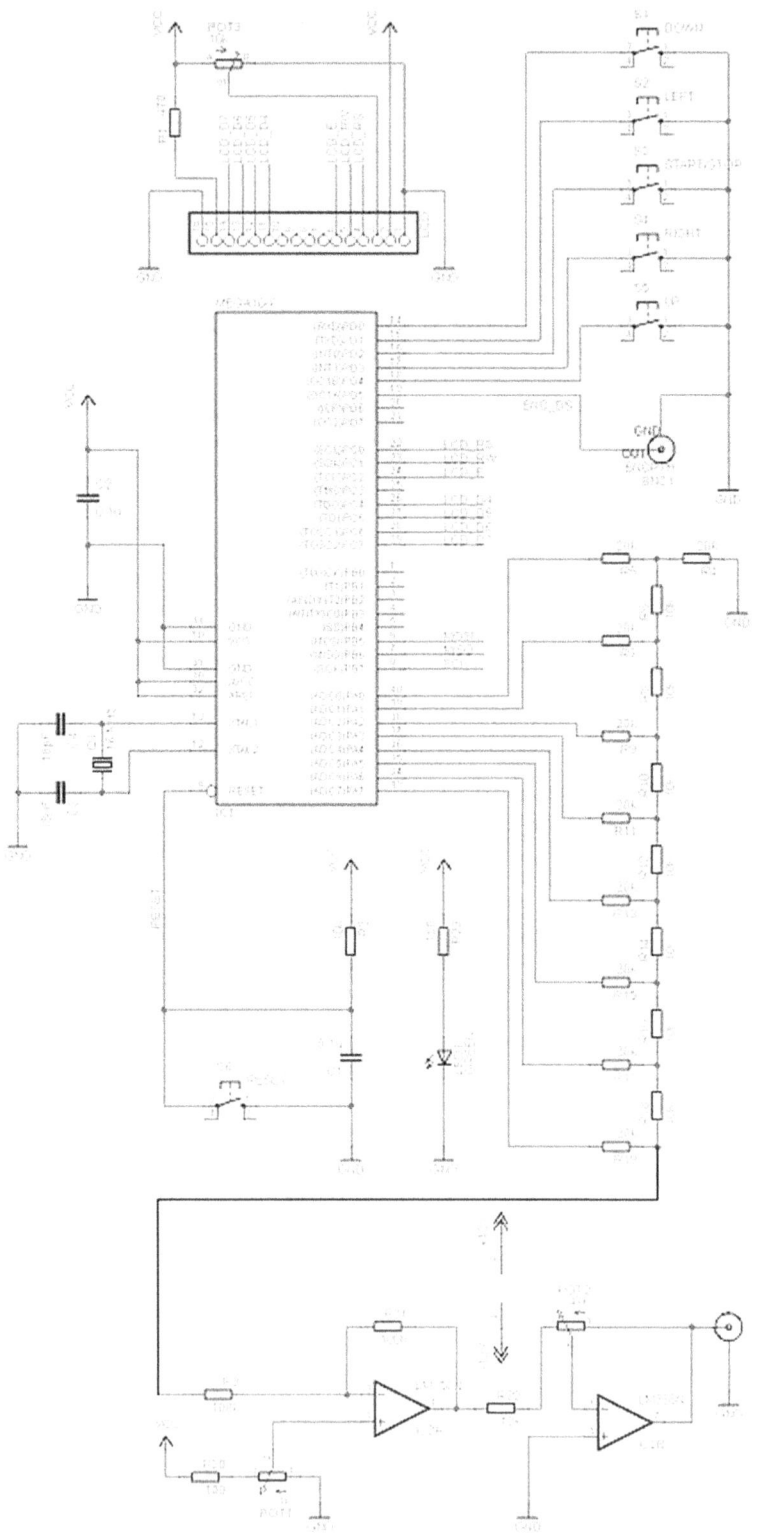

64

Here are the instructions that come with the function generator. I fixed up the English to make it more readable.

Specifications:
• Operating voltage: DC9-12V
• DDS frequency range: 1HZ-65534Hz.
• High-speed frequency (HS) output up to 8MHz;
• DDS signal amplitude and the offset amount can be adjusted separately by two potentiometers.
• DDS signals: sine wave, square wave, sawtooth, reverse sawtooth, triangle wave, ECG wave.
• 1602 LCD menu.
• Intuitive keyboard.
• Section rate steps: 1,10,100,1000,10000 Hz.
(How fast it steps when you push the right and left frequency up/down buttons)
• The power automatically restores the settings that were used the last time.
• Offset range: 0.5V pp to 5V pp
• Amplitude amount: 0.5V pp to 14V pp

Key Functions:
The UP button selects the waveform type
The DOWN button selects the waveform type
The LEFT button decreases the frequency
The RIGHT button increases the frequency
The START / STOP button turns the output waveform on and off
(In the off state, the "left "and "right" keys set the output frequency. The middle button starts and stops the selected waveform)

"UP" output waveforms selection order:
ECG = electrocardiogram wave
Rev Sawtooth = reverse sawtooth
SawTooth = sawtooth
Triangle = triangle wave
Square = square wave

There are also DDS sweep generators. These signal generators can be programmed to sweep through a range of frequencies. The DDS signal generator shown here is a model FY2100S.

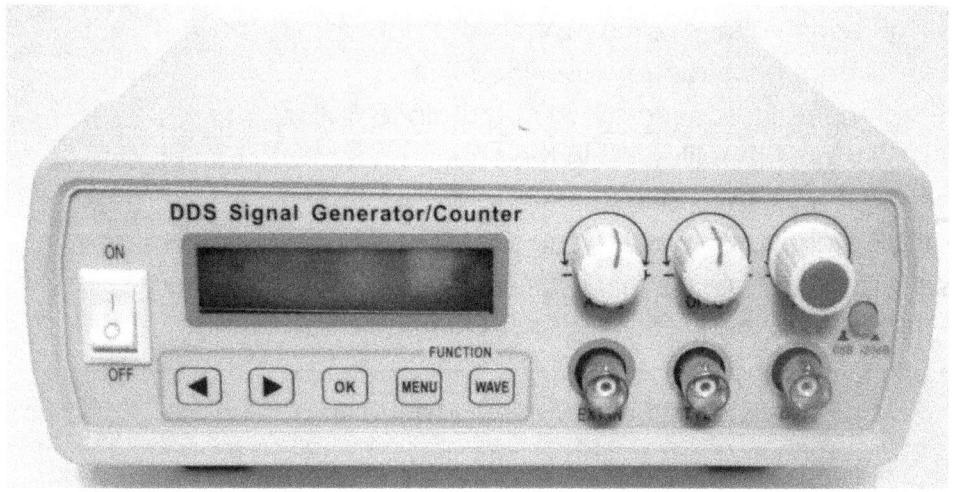

Some of its features include:
Waveforms: Sine, Square, and Triangle
Amplitude: up to (V peak to peak
DC Offset: + and – 2.5 Volts
Frequency Range: .01 Hz to 2 MHz.
Accuracy: + and – $1x10^{-6}$
Distortion: <.8% at 1KHz

Operation.
Use left and right arrows to select the digit to change
Use the right most knob to change the value of the selected digit
Use "OK" to change the range (usually Hz)
Use "Wave" to select waveform (Usually a sine wave)
  Then use arrows to select "Lin-Sweep: Stop"
  Then "OK" to change to "Run"

But first you will need to save your frequencies to M1 (Start frequency) and M2 (stop frequency). Otherwise it will either not run or run full the full range. To store the frequency use "menu" to highlight the bottom row. Then use the left and right arrows to get to "Func: Save". Then use the right knob to select the memory number. It will save whatever frequency is being displayed on the top line. When it is properly programmed going to "Lin-Sweep: Stop" (or Run) and pressing "OK" will cause it to start working. The display will count through the frequencies that are being generated. The next pictures shows a sweep of 300 Hz to 330 Hz being run.

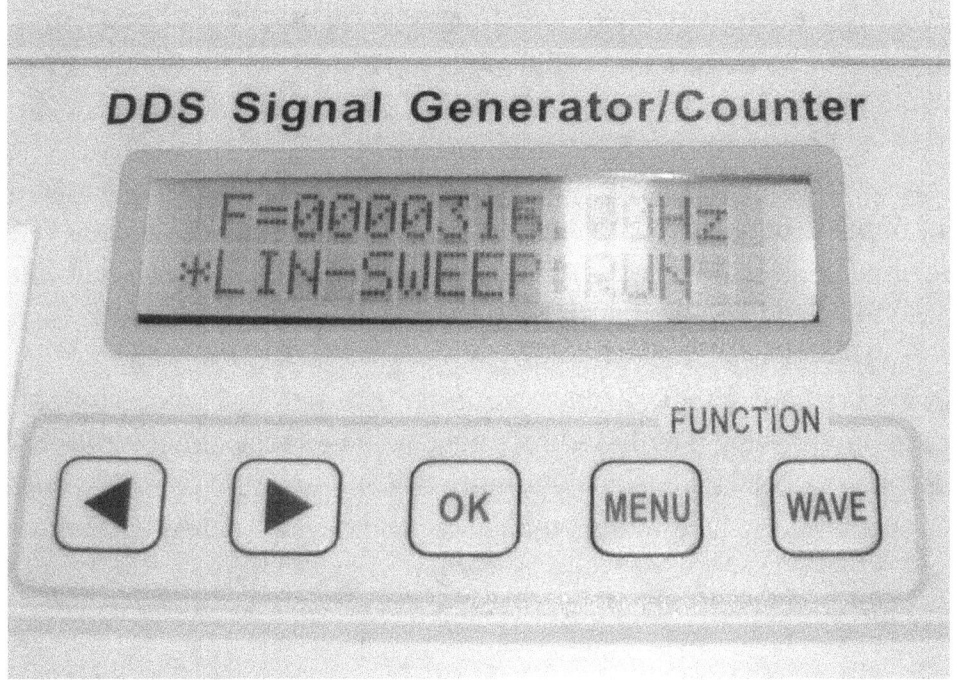

Chapter 13

Alternative Coil Designs

In my research on "Transcranial Magnetic Stimulation" I have discovered that there are some special types of coils that are usually used in order to concentrate the magnetic field.

I was looking for a way to make a more powerful coil as there was a lot of pain coming from my hips and none of the regular devices seemed able to help reduce that pain. Perhaps concentrating the magnetic field could be a solution to reaching deeper problems.

In the previous chapters we assumed a "Normal" coil type. Normal coils have evenly distributed magnetic fields usually concentrated around the coil itself. However there are two types of coils that can concentrate the field into a smaller area. They are called "Butterfly" or "Figure 8" coils. Some articles seem to say that these two types are the same thing, but I beg to differ.

Butterfly coils are two coils that sometimes overlap each other slightly. The result is a magnetic field that is twice (or more) powerful under the overlapped area. Some butterfly coils do not overlap and still have a concentrated field under the area that is closest to the area where the coils are closest to each other.

This next drawing shows first a side view then, below that, it shows a top view of the coils.

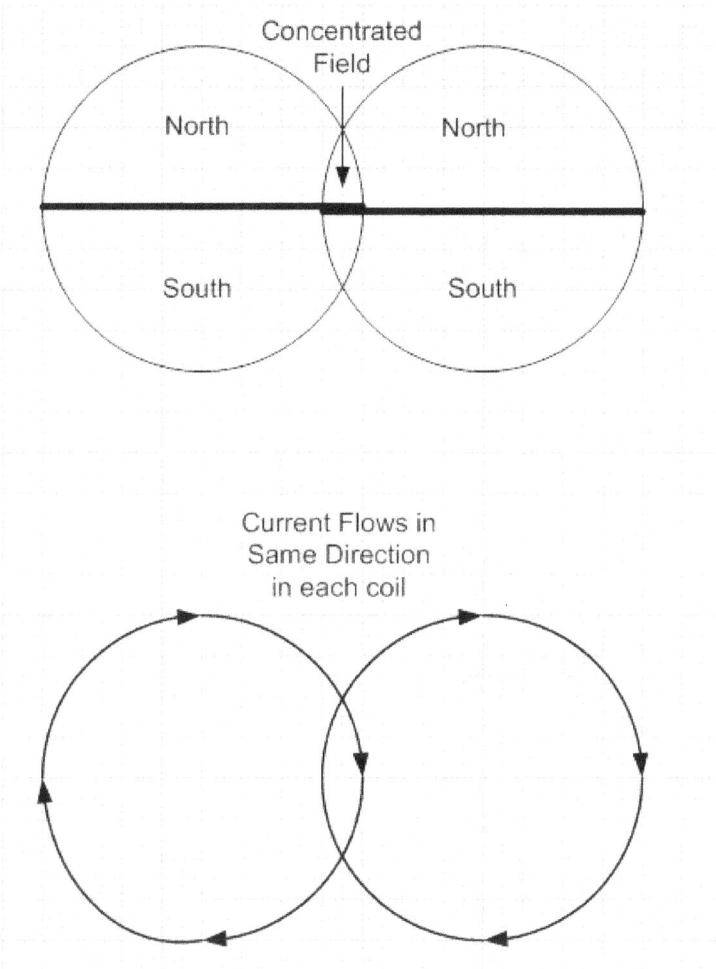

Figure 8 coils look the same, but the two coils are wired with opposing polarity. That is because in a figure 8 the wires on each half of the 8 rotate in the opposite direction thus producing a magnetic field that is reversed in each half of the coil assembly.

This results in two unusual things. One change is that the fields have to pull back from each other so the resulting two magnetic fields are not perfectly round. The second thing is that the induced magnetic fields are North for one coil and South for the other coil resulting in essentially an induced current flowing between the two concentration points.

In the next drawing the top illustration is a side view of the coils and the bottom drawing is a top view of the coils.

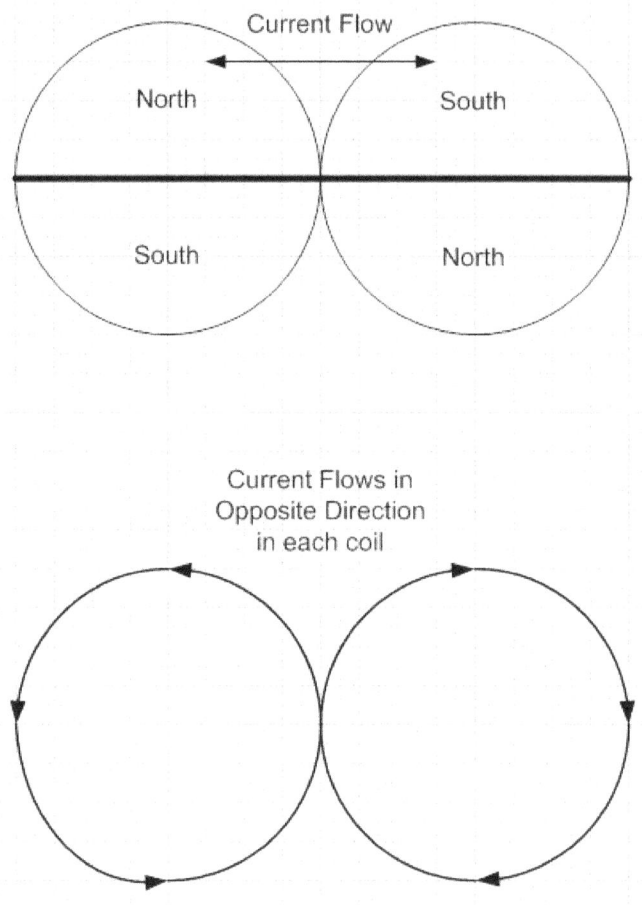

One way to make a Figure 8 coil is to make a "normal" coil on a trash can or whatever, them twist it so that it forms a figure 8. Here is a picture of a home made figure 8 coil made out of 18 gauge wire from a TV set degausing coil. The degaussing coil was first rewound onto a trach can then slid off and then it was twisted. Then it was wrapped in electrical tape to insulate it.

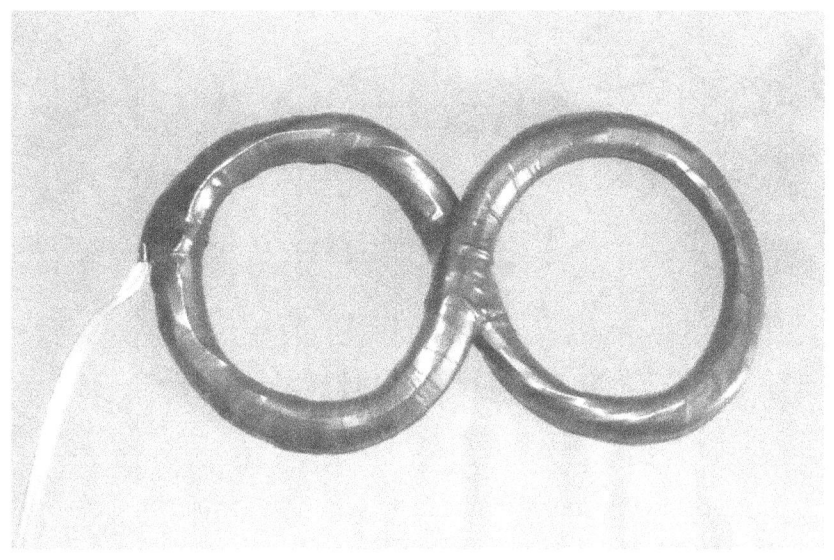

This type of figure 8 coil could be used with a low power "Doug" coil. To use it with a "Thumper" type of coil a larger wire gauge should be used.

To make a figure 8 thumper coil I think two one inch diameter dowels fastened to a piece of plywood about 5 inches apart might do. You could then wind the wire in a figure 8. Then you would have to pry the resulting coil off the form and wrap it in electrical tape.

Chapter 14

Tesla Coil,

High voltage and Ozone

Most people do not know that before Tesla invented our power grid, Tesla was actually trying to improve people's health with is electronic devices. The ozone that is generated by his coils was supposed to improve the health of people.

There are several common types of Tesla coils.

1. Fixed spark gap
2. Rotary spark gap
3. Vacuum tube
4. Solid state

I started playing with Tesla coils when I was only in my teens. I planned on zapping my brother so he would never walk into my room without knocking again. I wired it up to the doorknob and turned it on. Someone knocked on my door, so I turned everything off and opened the door. My sister was standing there, she wanted to know what I was doing that was causing every TV and Radio in the house to go crazy.

My first Tesla coil design used cardboard forms from Christmas wrapping paper, and rewound degaussing coils removed from old TV's. For a High Voltage power transformer I used a 6KV transformer that was used to light some sort of Neon tube. The spark gap was just two sewing needles facing each other. The capacitor was a sheet of plastic with aluminum foil on each side. I tried to use that Tesla coil to try to keep my annoying little brother from walking into my room without knocking!

My biggest Tesla coil is a type of fixed spark gap that is called a "multi gap". The spark gap is cooled by a 110 Volt fan. This is an earlier picture of the Tesla coil showing the two foot long sparks coming off the top load.

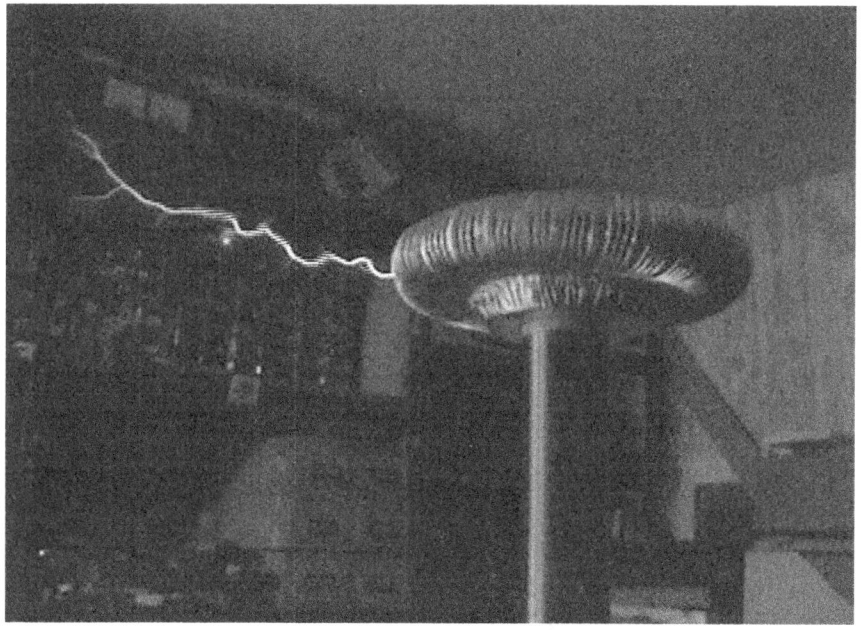

The primary coil is 12 turns 10 gauge insulated copper wire with an inside diameter of five inches and an outside diameter of 12 inches. The secondary is about 1000 turns wound on a two foot long piece of three inch diameter PVC. The top load is two aluminum pie pans that are glued together. Then a flexible aluminum dryer vent pipe is wrapped around the pie plates and glued together. On the last run had it producing sparks well over two feet long. They were twice as long as they were when I was using a 10 KV 25 ma OBIT transformer.

Below is a picture of the "guts" of my big Tesla coil. The part in front center is the safety gap. On each side of the safety gap are the choke coils. Between the two choke coils is the high voltage capacitor and behind that is the air cooled multi spark gap with the black cooling fan on the right side. The power transformer is not seen in the picture, it was sitting on the ground. The power transformer is an Actown 12 KV 30 MA NST or Neon Sign Transformer. It cost me around $50.00 to buy it on eBay.

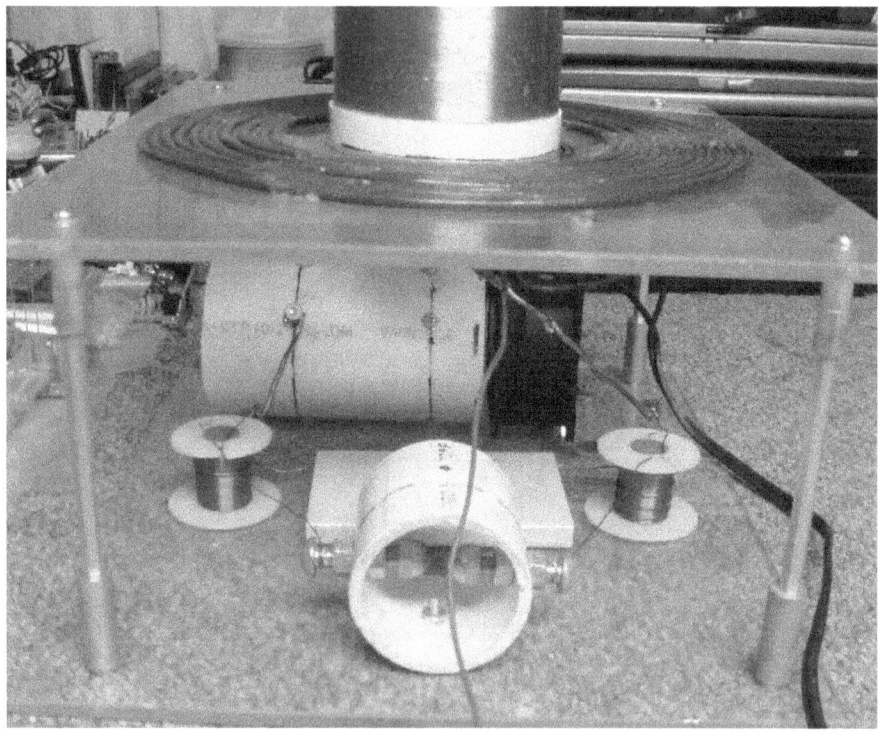

Up next is a picture looking through the PVC pipe to see the multiple spark gaps that are made from four inch pieces of Copper pipe. It is air cooled by a 110 volt fan located at the far end. Eventually another copper pipe was added.

You can see the large yellow high voltage capacitor to the right of the spark gap. An earlier design used a .0053 at 15KV Door Knob Capacitor that I had purchased on eBay.

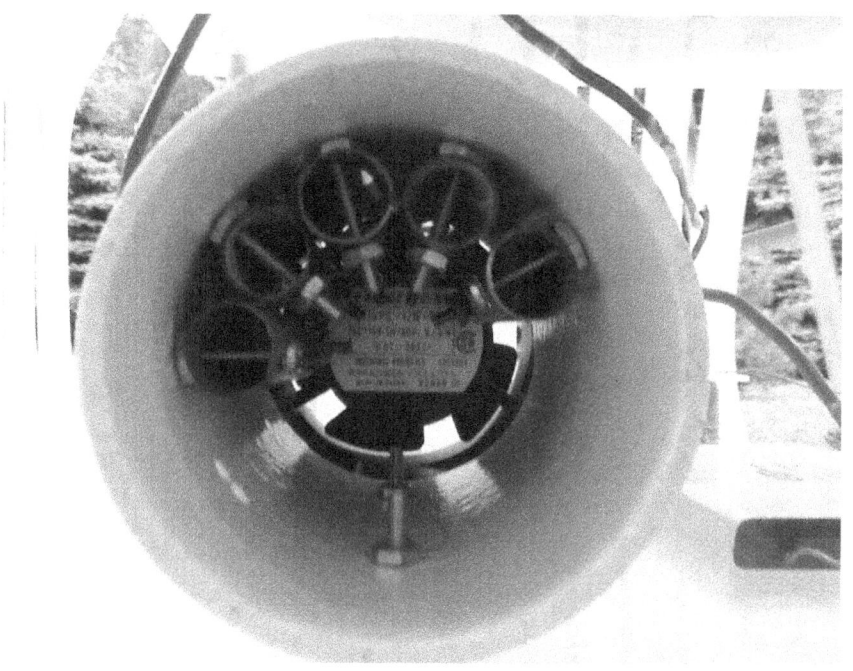

The top load of my Tesla coil is an aluminum pie plate with a flexible aluminum metal drier vent pipe wrapped around it. It can then be covered with some aluminum duct tape to get a smoother surface. Below is a picture of some home made top loads. Two aluminum pie plates glued together might also work.

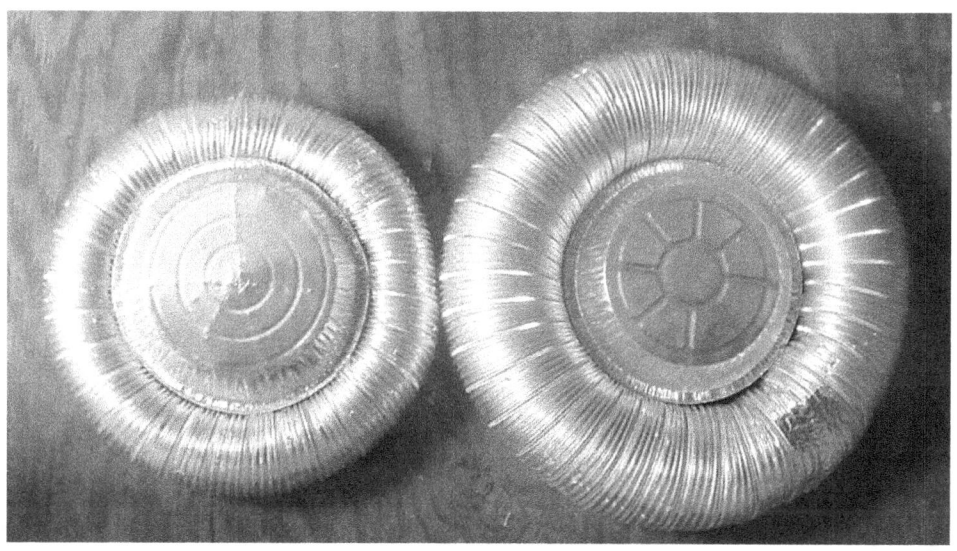

Up next is the schematic of my biggest Tesla coil. For proper operation a good ground connection is needed. Ideally the ground should be connected to a metal ground rod. The schematic diagram does not show the 110 volt cooling fan.

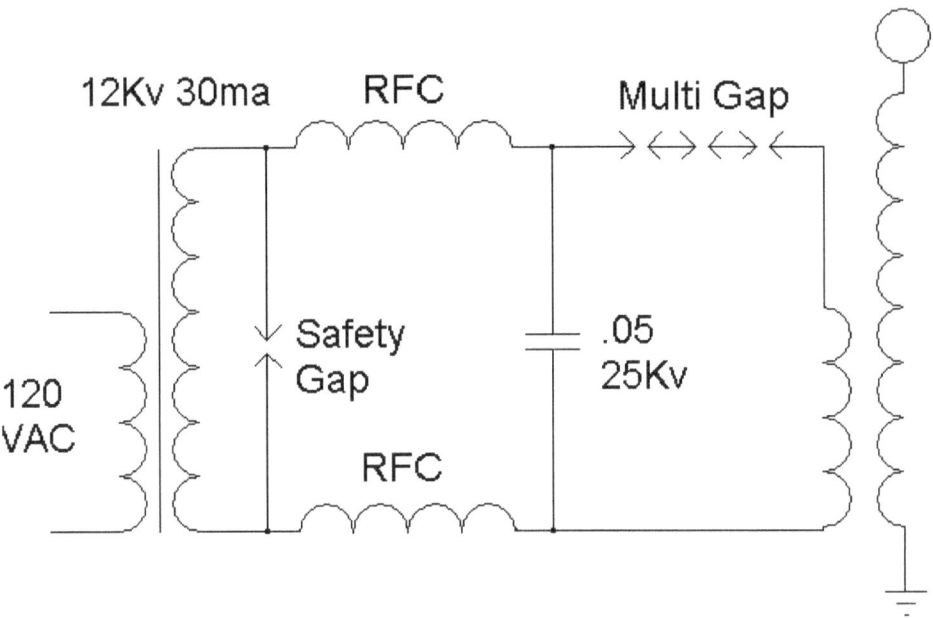

Parts list for Tesla coil.
1 – 12 Kv 30 ma high voltage power transformer
1 – ½ inch adjustable safety gap
2 – Radio Frequency Chokes – may be from speaker crossovers
1 - .05 mF at 25 KV paper capacitor
1 – Multi gap made of ½ inch copper pipes at around .1 inch spacing
1 – Primary coil of 10 gauge wire (see text)
1 – Secondary coil of 1000 turns 18 gauge enameled wire on a three inch form
1 – Three inch square 110 volt cooling fan
1 – Top load (Pie pan with dryer vent)

Chapter 15

Vacuum Tube Tesla Coil

A vacuum tube Tesla coil replaces the spark gap with a vacuum tube to switch the power on and off to the coil. Vacuum tubes are usually worked beyond their normal safe limits in Tesla Coils. For instance the 812 tube is rated for about 800 volts but it is being run at 2000 volts for this Tesla coil.

I do not think that vacuum tube Tesla coils produce nearly as much ozone as spark gap types. Also, in my opinion, they are much more dangerous to operate as they operate with a higher input power as far as current is concerned.

The plate of the one tube Tesla coil glows red hot while it is running. If two tubes are used there should be less of a strain on the tubes. Using two tubes will add more power as well. The two tube version will even use two Microwave oven transformers for more power and a full wave rectifier for less AC on the output. Another advantage of using two microwave oven transformers is that the filament voltage of 6 volts can be reached by connecting the two 3 volt windings already on the transformers together. The primaries should be wired out of phase and the 3 volt windings in series to reach the needed 6 volts for the tubes to light up.

The two tube Tesla coil has burned up several times while the design was being perfected. There were problems with arcs between the grid and the plate coils, as well as between the plate coil and the secondary coil. The grid coil was eventually replaced with 20 turns of #18 about 3/4 of an inch below the plate coil. This resolved arcs from the grid coil to the plate coil. The secondary coil was raised up about 1 inch to reduce the amount of high voltage present close to the plate coil. A bigger plate coil, perhaps using a 5 or 6 inch diameter form would be a better solution. I also am only using the 2KV from one transformer.

Below is a picture of the dual 812 vacuum tube Tesla coil. The output sparks are not nearly as long as the spark gap types of Tesla coils but they are really more intense and they are hot enough to even melt the end of the wire! I put a nail at the end of the wire so it would not melt the wire. The nail gets hot enough to melt plastic.

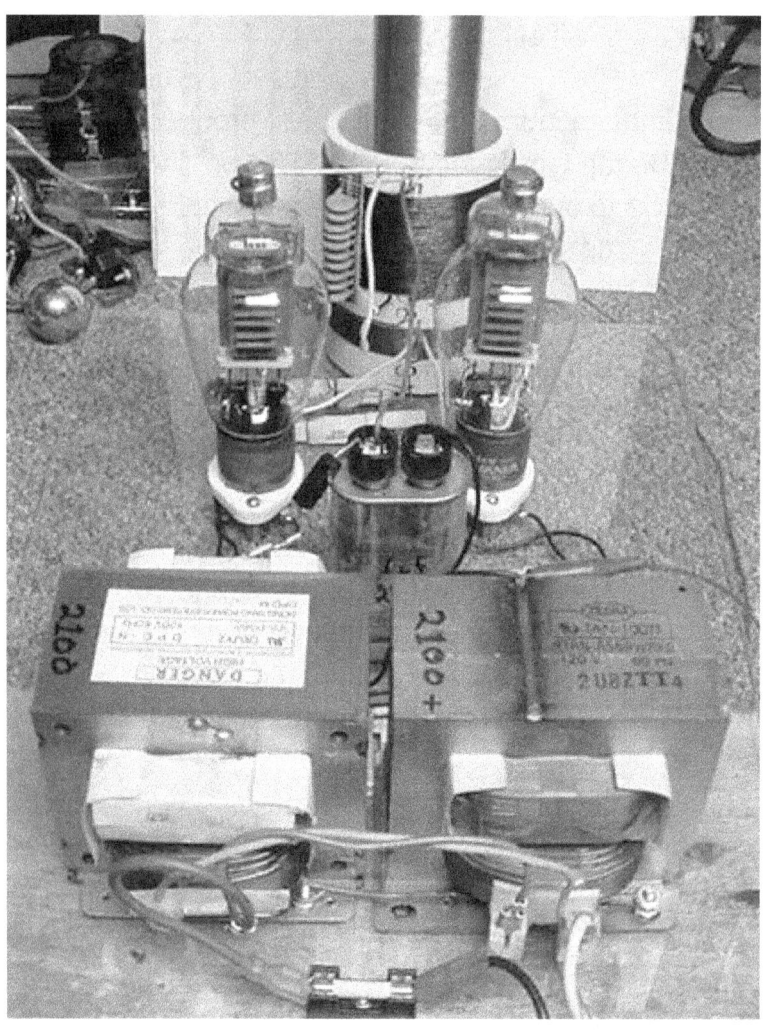

Here is the schematic diagram of the dual vacuum tube Tesla coil.
I usually connected only one of the 2 KV transformer windings.
That was to reduce the power going through the vacuum tubes.

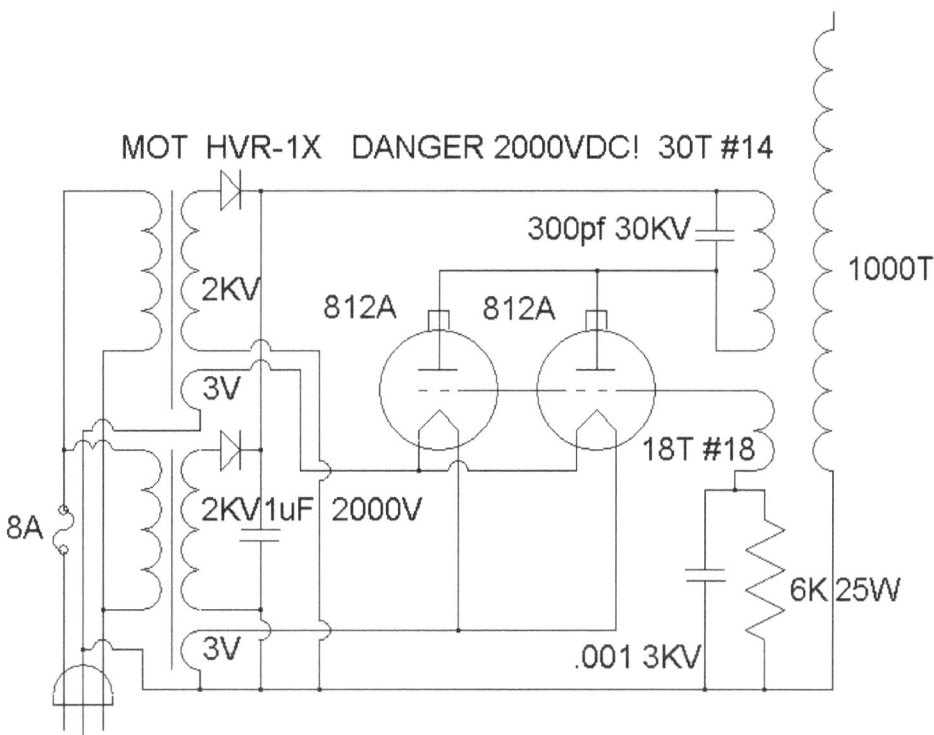

Parts list for dual vacuum tube Tesla coil:
2 – Microwave oven transformers
1 – 8 amp fuse and holder
2 – Microwave oven diodes
1 – 2uF 2000 volt microwave oven capacitor
2 – 812A vacuum tubes and 4 pin sockets
1 - .001 3KV ceramic capacitor
1 – 300 pf 30 KV ceramic capacitor (3 x .001 capacitors in series)
1 – 6K 25 watt power resistor (or 6 x 10 watt resistors in series)
1 – Primary coil on a 3 inch form 18 turns #18 and 30 turns #14 one half inch apart.
1 – Secondary coil on a 1.5 inch form about 1000 turns 18 gauge enameled wire.

Chapter 16

Aluminum Washer Launcher

While playing with the super thumper, I noticed that it could make an aluminum washer bounce. By making the coil smaller, I could get the washer to fly several inches up into the air. I kept making the coil smaller and smaller. Then I decided to wind a totally flat coil. That is not an easy thing to do. I even developed my own coil form using a five inch square piece of wood with a rotating 3/4 inch piece of wood on top. I wound two or three turns of the coil then glued it down. Then, the next day, I would wind another two or three turns then glue them. Eventually I made a totally flat coil about 5.5 inches in diameter. With that coil I was able to put dents in the ceiling since the washers now flew over 8 feet high.

Coming up next is a picture of the flat coil being made; it is not easy to do.

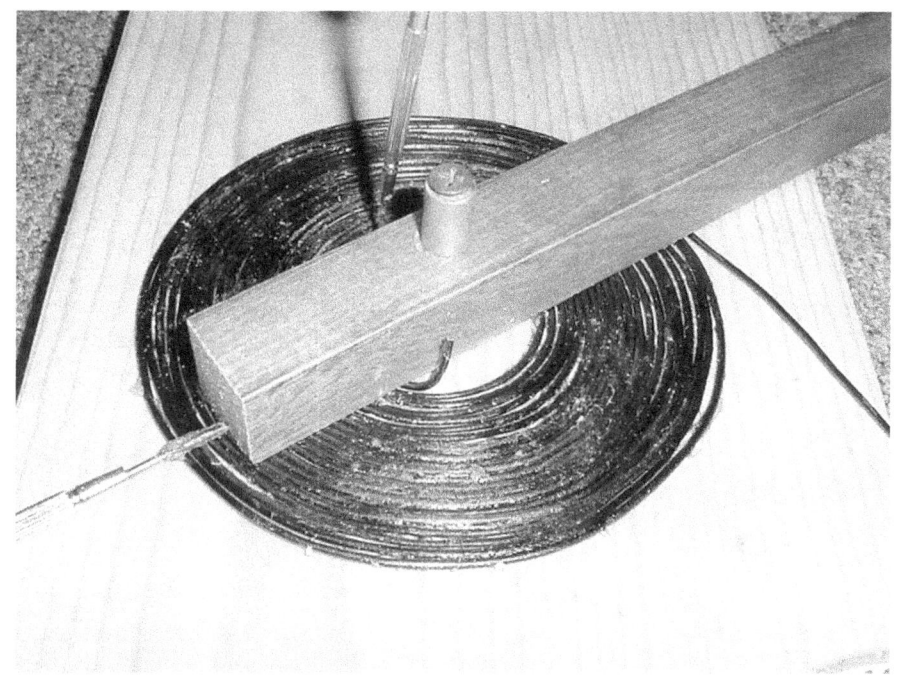

The next thing I did was to make a bigger power supply. I went from using 300 volts to 900 volts. The power supply used a microwave transformer that I had center tapped to get about 1KV. Then I had four big 250 volt capacitors that came out of old telephone systems power supplies. I continued to use a stud mounted SCR until I fried it. With this power supply a 5.5 inch washer, made out of an old hard drive, would fly about 20 to 25 feet straight up.

The next picture is of the 900 volt power supply. The SCR was way in the back. The meter goes across the capacitors. The right meter does not work.

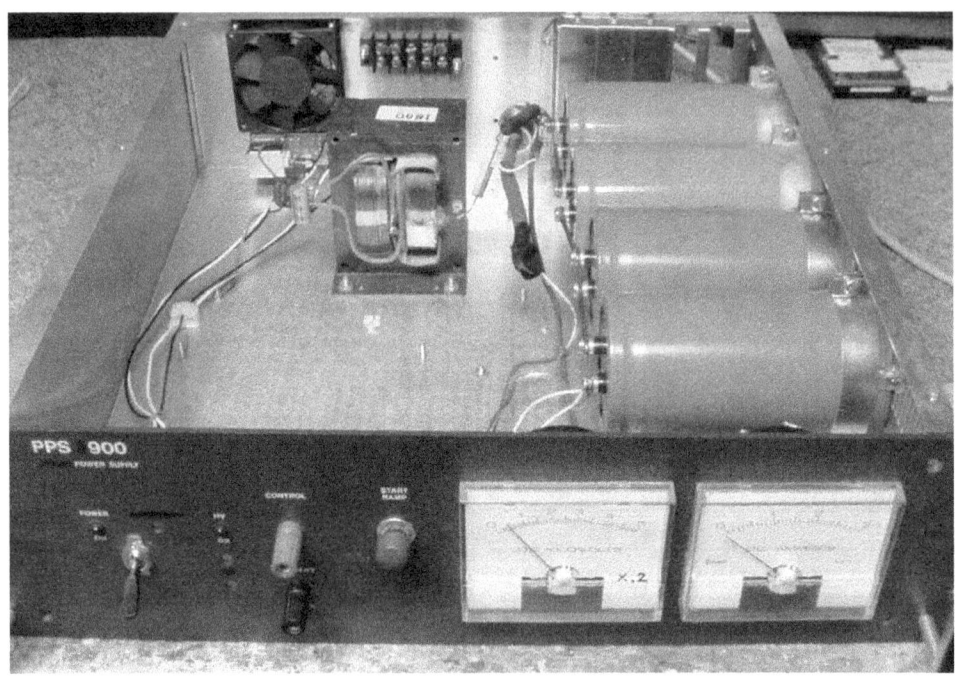

Up next is the schematic diagram of the 900 volt power supply for the washer launcher.

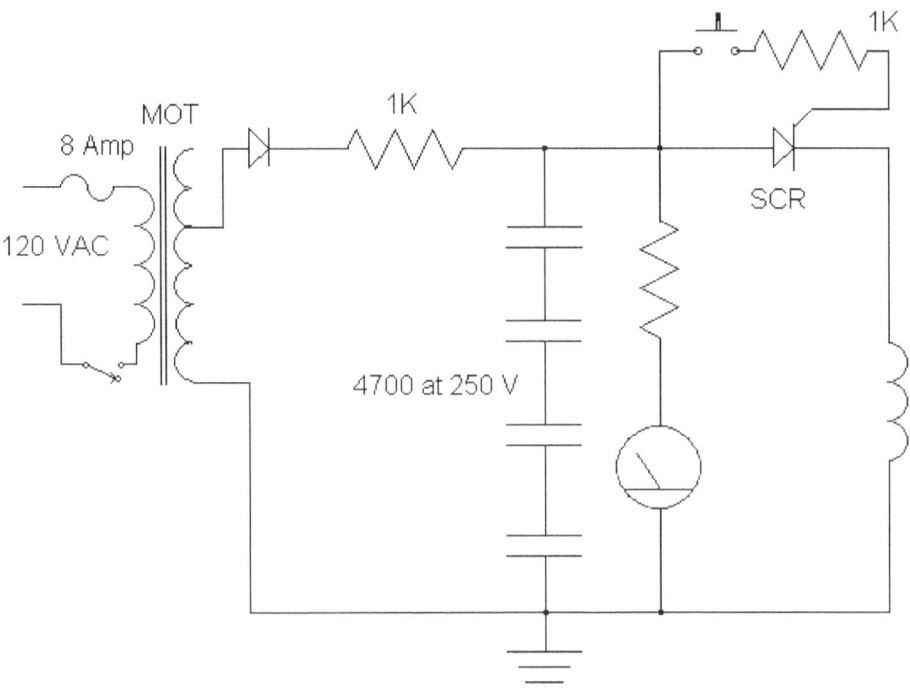

Parts list for 900 volt power supply:

1 -- 8 amp fuse and socket

1 – Power switch

1 – Power Jack

1 – Center tapped microwave oven power transformer

1 – Microwave oven diode

1 – 1K 50 watt power resistor

4 – 4700 uF at 250 volt capacitors

1 -- Momentary contact well insulated switch

1 – Very big SCR

1 – 1K ½ watt resistor

1 – Meter capable of 1 KV.

1 – Flat coil

2 – Banana jacks and plugs.

Did I stop there? Nope! At the Rochester HamFest I purchased a box full of 5700 at 400 volt (450 volt peak) capacitors. Now I could step up to using 1600 volts. At this point the SCR blew and I replaced it with a "Block" Thyristor device. The ED431825 Thyristor can handle up to 1,800 volts and 6,500 amps.

Here are the thyristor's specifications:

Part Number = ED431825

Manufacturer Name = Powerex Power Semiconductors

Description = SCR Doubler Module

V(DRM) Max.(V)Rep. Peak Off Volt. = 1.8k

V(RRM) Max. (V) = 1.8k

I(T) Max.(A) On-state Current = 250±

I(TSM) Max. (A) = 6.5k

     at t(w) (s) (Test Condition) = 8.3m

I(GT) Max. (A) = 150m

V(GT) Max.(V) = 3

I(D) Max. (A) Leakage Current = 50m

     at Temp. (°C) (Test Condition) = 130

V(T) Max. (V) = 1.3

at I(T) (A) (Test Condition) = 625
dv/dt Min. (V/us) = 500
T(q) Typ. (s) = 150u
T(gt) Typ. (s) = 150u

Here is a picture of the 1600 volt power supply. This time there are two banks of capacitors in parallel. The second power transformer was not in use. I used the banana plugs to attach the coil at first. However they quickly melted down, so I had to use binding posts to connect the coil to the power supply in later versions.

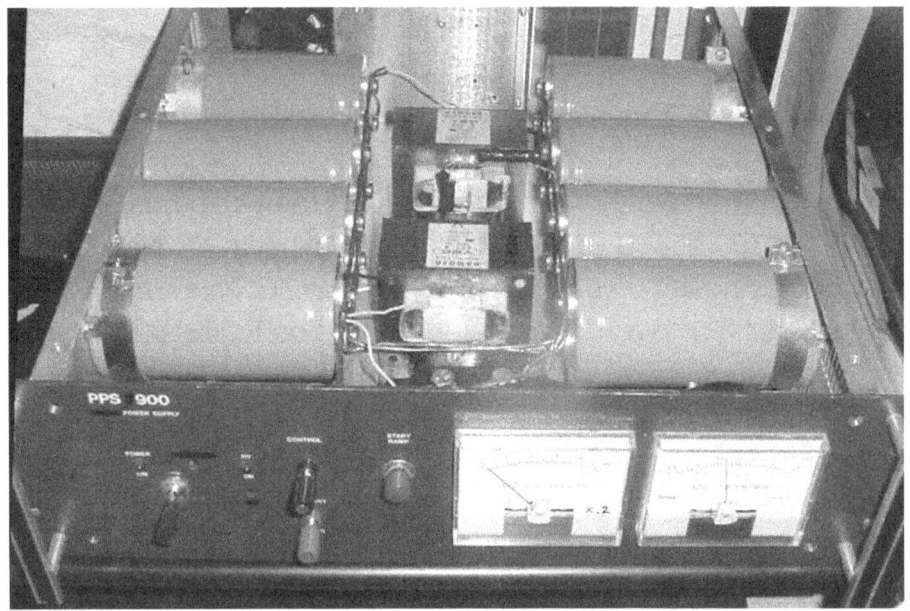

The next picture is a close up view of the guts of the 1600 volt power supply.

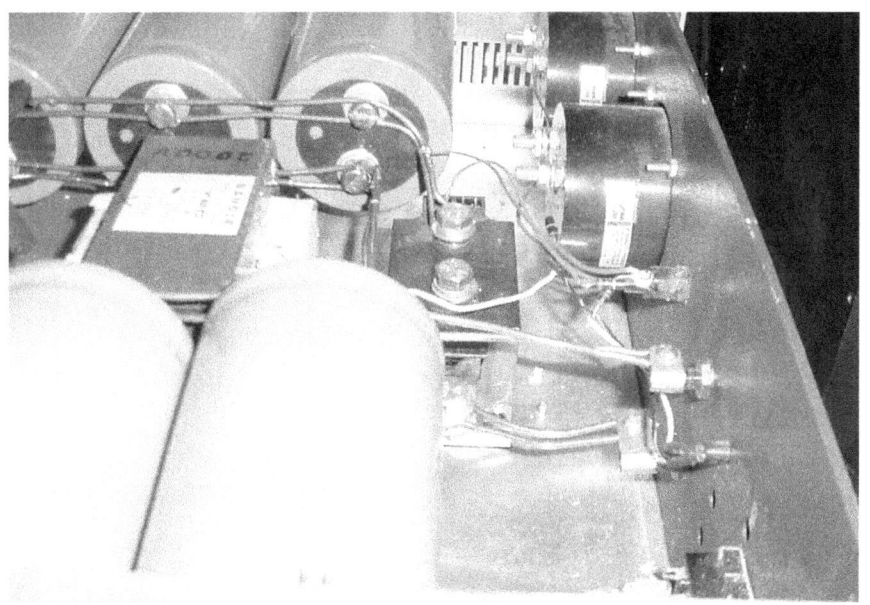

Below is the schematic diagram of the 1600 volt power supply.

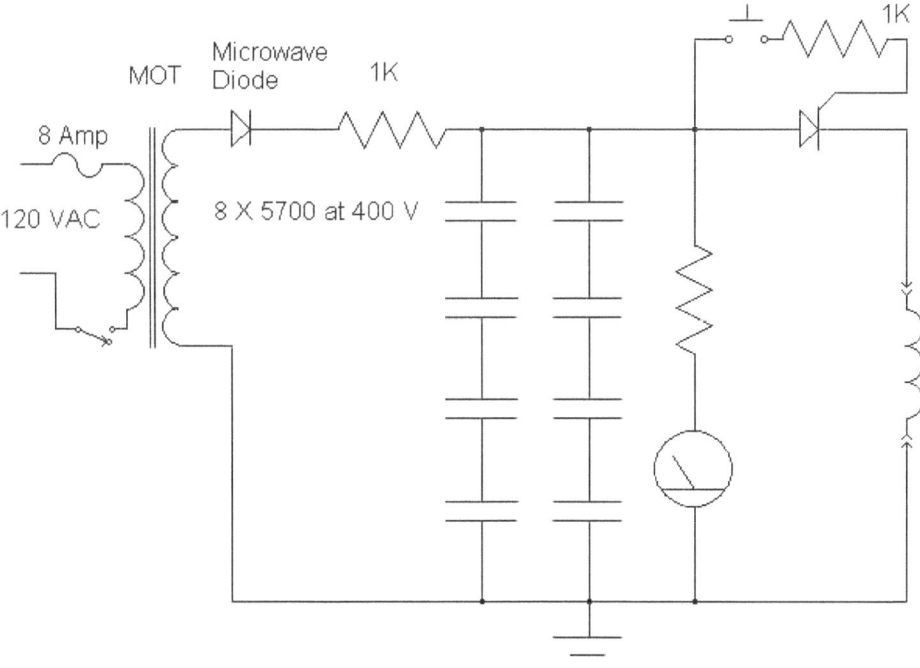

Here is a parts list for 1600 volt power supply:

1 -- 8 amp fuse and socket
1 – Power switch
1 – Power Jack
1 – Microwave oven power transformer
1 – Microwave oven diode
1 – 1K 50 watt power resistor
8 – 5700 uF at 400 volt (450V surge) capacitors
1 -- Momentary contact well insulated switch
1 – ED431825 1,800 Volt Thyristor
1 – 1K ½ watt resistor
1 – Meter capable of 2 KV.
1 – Flat coil
2 – Banana jacks and plugs.

Around this time I started setting a soda can on top of the washer. Then, above that, I would place a cinder block that was held up by bricks. When it was fired the soda can was then crushed up against the cinder block. The soda can would end up nearly flat!

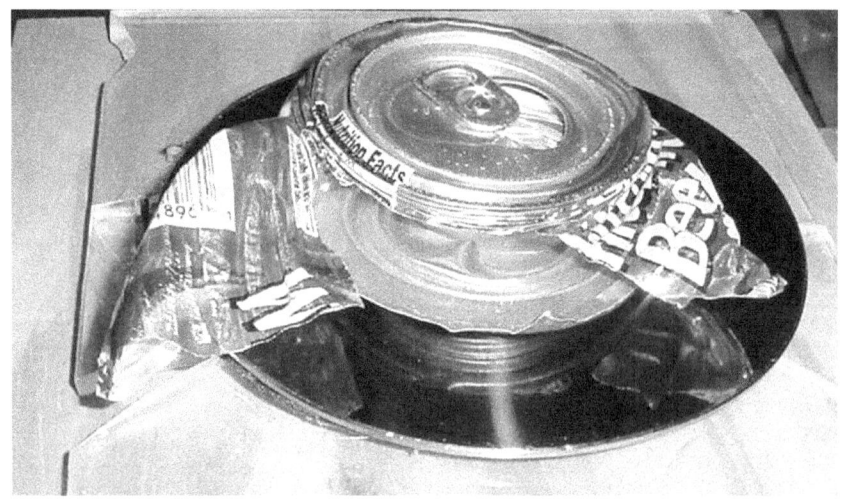

There a several video's of the washer launcher in operation on YouTube. The washers were flying about 35 feet through the air in some of the videos. I have also used the aluminum washer launcher to destroy a pumpkin, snowman, and various other things.

Chapter 17

Soda Can Crusher

Did I stop at 1600 volts? Of course not! Next up was a 5000 volt power supply that I purchased on eBay. I purchased what was called a "Gas Puff Valve" on eBay. It featured a mechanical contactor that could handle almost anything. However, I quickly fried the power supply that came with it on the first test firing, and then I took out the capacitor on the second test run.

I was afraid that the flat coil that I had been using could not take any more than 1600 volts, as the coil would deform whenever it was used at that voltage. So I switched to a coil that wraps around the soda can instead. It was made out of four or five turns of 10 or 12 gauge electrical wire.

Coming up next is a picture of the high voltage contactor and the coil that goes over the soda can.

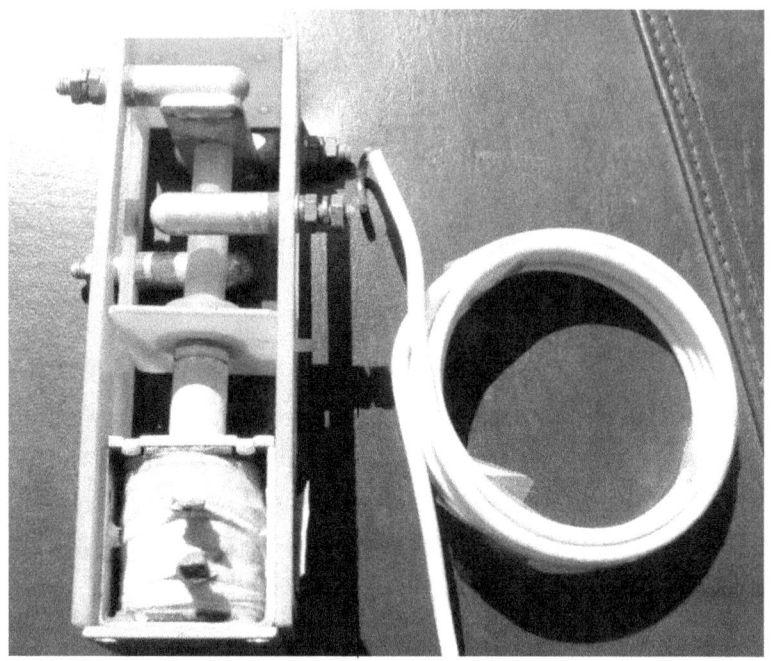

This next picture is what the complete "Gas Puff Valve" assembly looked like when I first received it. You can see the round capacitor in the back left corner. The contactor is in the back center. The glass meter cover (front left side) was shattered, but the meter still worked.

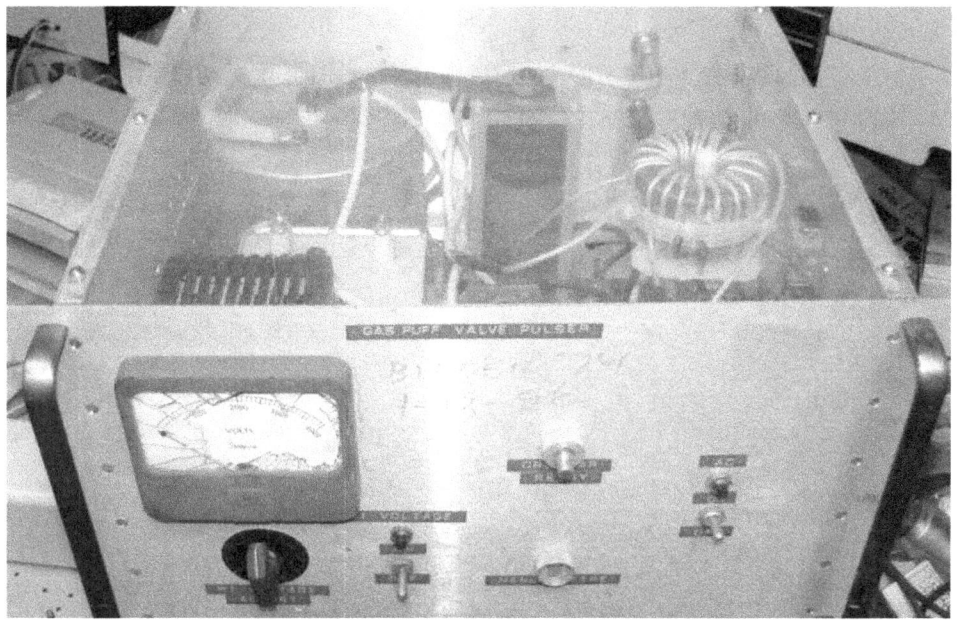

I replaced the blown capacitor with a deliberator capacitor. The blown power transformer was replaced with a microwave oven power transformer and voltage doubler consisting of a capacitor and two high voltage diodes. Coming up next is the schematic diagram of the rebuilt 5 KV power supply. The new capacitor was rated at 20 uF at 5KV.

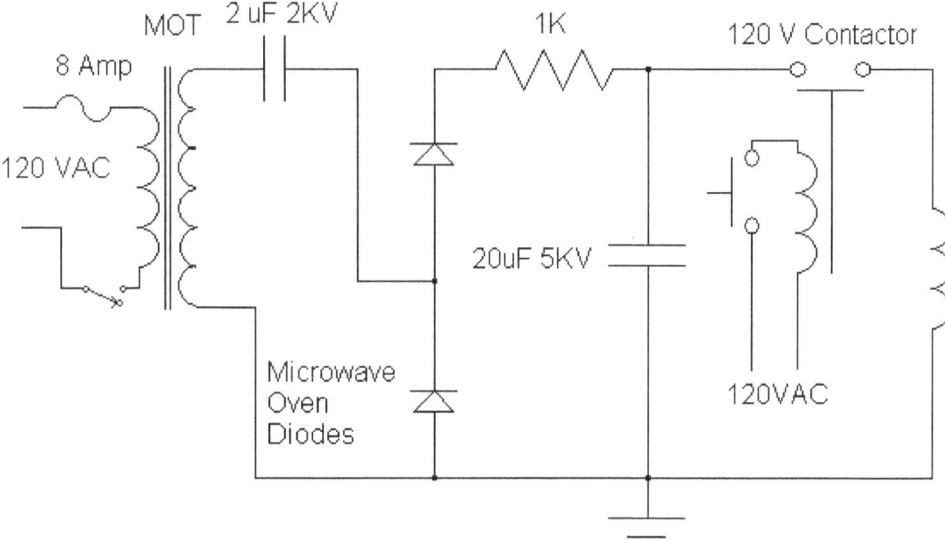

The next picture is what the can crusher looked like when it was operating. You can see smoke rising out of the soda can.

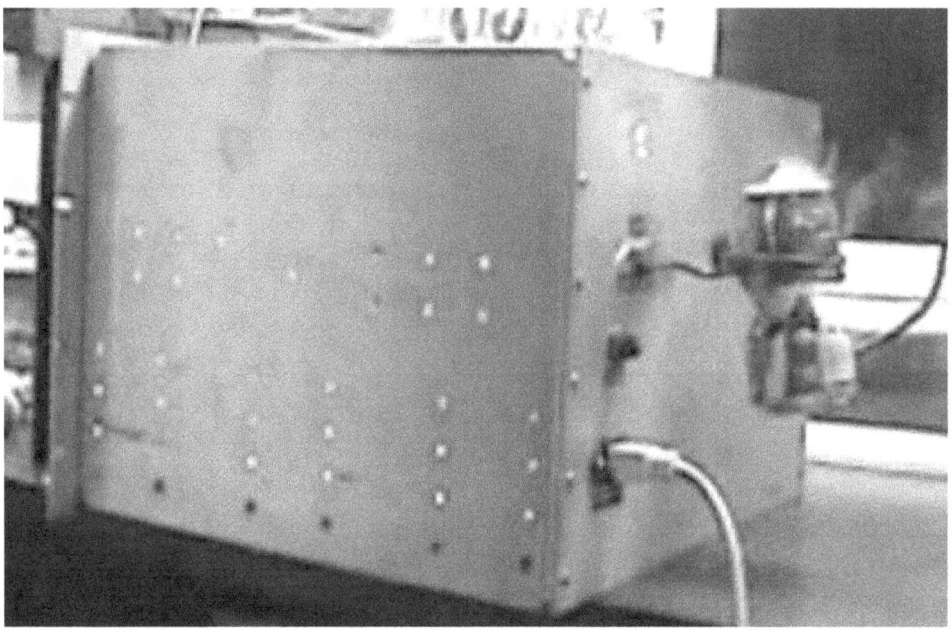

This next picture shows what it does to a soda can when it is fired. It can almost completely cut the soda can in half!

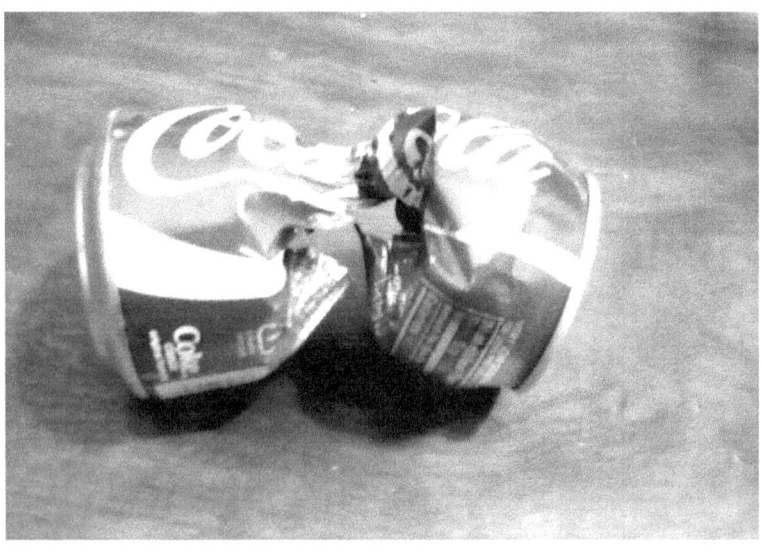

Chapter 18

Magnetic Coil Gun

At some point I also wound a coil around a piece of 1/2 inch diameter plastic pipe. The coil was made out of three layers of 20 turns each of 14 gauge enameled wire. Each layer was wound then it was glued in place. The next day I would then wind the next layer. First a bolt with a nut on it was placed in the tube and then 300 volts DC from the "super thumper" was applied to the coil. The bolt would fly out of the pipe with enough force to send a soda can flying. I adjusted the position of the coil on the tube to get the most launching power.

Here is a picture of that coil as it was being made.

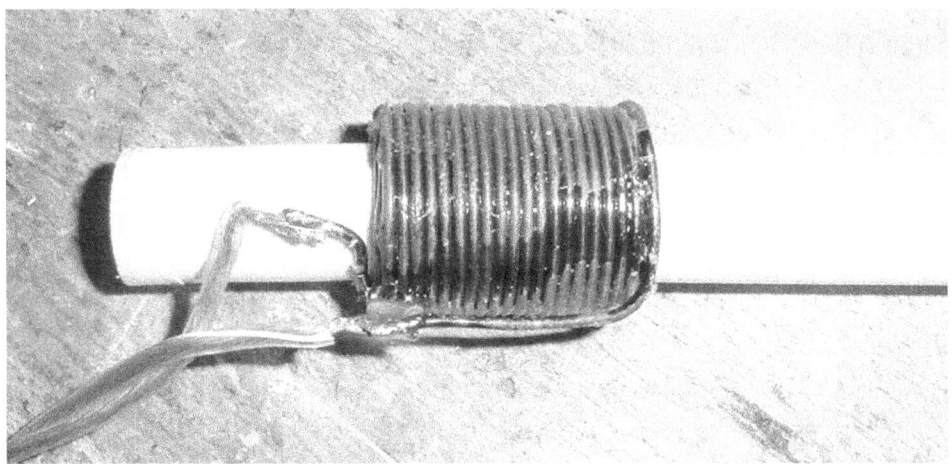

Up next is another picture of the coil gun that also shows the 1/2 inch bolt. I used a nut to balance the bolt. The bolt is the correct length that when it is bottomed in the tube so the end of the bolt is just inside of the coil it will fire with the most power.

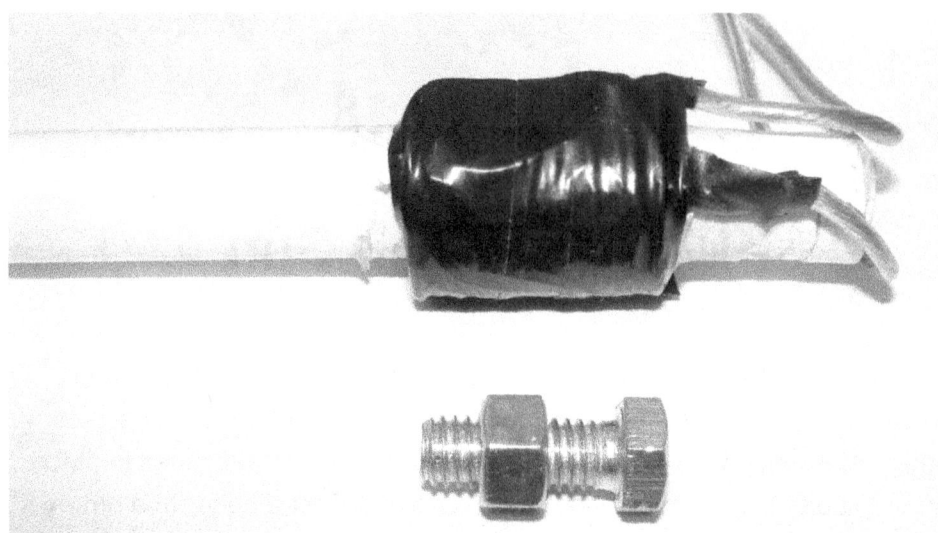

For my next coil gun, I wound an almost identical coil on an empty pen shell the size of a typical pencil. This time the inside diameter of the coil was only about that 1/4 of an inch in diameter. This coil consisted of five layers of about 25 turns each. Again each layer of the coil was wound then glued into place before the next layer was wound.

Then a larger finishing nail with a small head was placed so that the tip of the nail was just inside of the coil. When power was applied, the nail would fly out of the other side of the coil with enough force to penetrate clear through a soda can. There was a cinder block located behind the soda can to stop the nail, just in case.

I never used more than 300 volts to fire the two coil guns. I was afraid that either the coil would damage the power supply or the power supply would damage the coil. However I did shoot several videos of the coil guns in action and then uploaded them to YouTube.

Coming up next is a picture of the second coil gun.

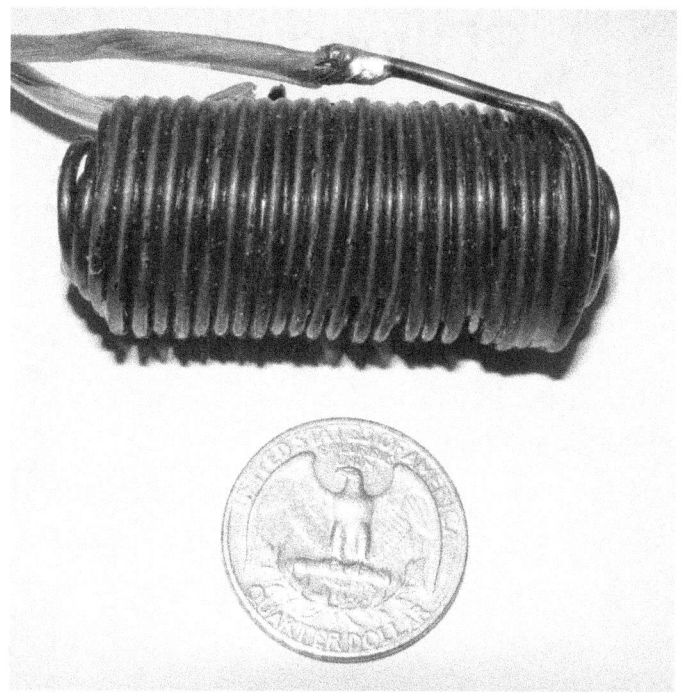

This next picture was extracted from one of the videos.

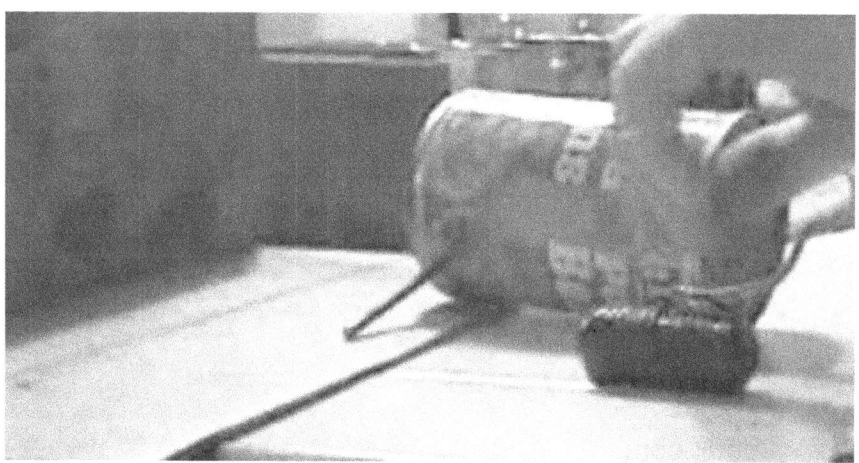

Bibliography

The cure for all diseases
By Hulda Clark
Copyright 1995
New Century Press
1055 Bay Blvd
Suite C
Chula Vista California 91911
www.newcenturypress.com

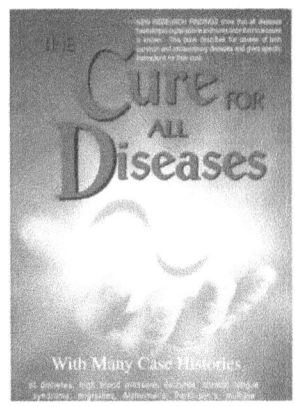

The Cure for all Caners

By Hulda Clark
Copyright 1992
New Century Press
1055 Bay Blvd
Suite C
Chula Vista California 91911
www.newcenturypress.com

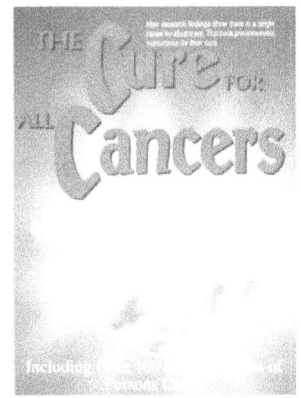

Lyme Disease and Rife Machines
By Bryan Rosner
Copyright 2004 by Bryan Rosner
www.lymebook.com

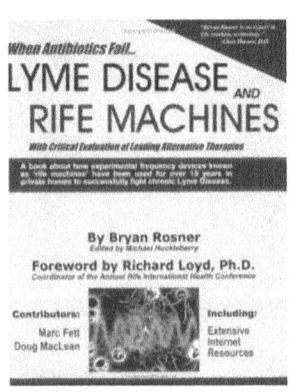

Other web sources:

www.royalrife.com

http://keelynet.com/biology/thumind.htm

www.newmediaexplorer.org/chris/2009/02/19/build_a_low_cost_si
mple_magnetic_pulser.htm <- This site has schematics

http://w5jgv.com/rife/2011_Rife_Beam-Ray_System/index.htm

https://www.slideserve.com/briar/lyme-disease-rife-machines

https://rifevideos.com/chapter_10_the_gruner_schematic_and_phili
p_hoylands_beam_ray_laboratory_rife_machine.html

http://spectrotek.com/

https://guruhq.com/how-to-build-a-rife-machine/